T0068181

TRAINING FOR LIFE

TRAINING FOR LIFE

*Wellness and Working Out with
Personal Trainers in Your Sixties
and Beyond*

DAVID E. LAPIN

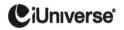

TRAINING FOR LIFE

WELLNESS AND WORKING OUT WITH PERSONAL TRAINERS IN YOUR SIXTIES AND BEYOND

iUniverse books may be ordered through booksellers or by contacting:

iUniverse
1663 Liberty Drive
Bloomington, IN 47403
www.iuniverse.com
844-349-9409

ISBN: 978-1-6632-5598-3 (sc)
ISBN: 978-1-6632-5597-6 (e)

Library of Congress Control Number: 2023916884

Print information available on the last page.

iUniverse rev. date: 09/13/2023

CONTENTS

Preface vii

Chapter 1   No Excuses 1

Chapter 2   True Believer 7

Chapter 3   Proprioception 13

Chapter 4   Storm Clouds 19

Chapter 5   Transition 25

Chapter 6   "Cat, Cow" 31

Chapter 7   Contrasts 37

Chapter 8   Fight Club 43

Chapter 9   Winter Walks 49

Chapter 10   Solitary Confinement 55

Chapter 11   A Deep Chill 61

Chapter 12   Welcome Reboots 67

Chapter 13   Risk/Reward 73

Chapter 14   A Lunch Date 79

Chapter 15   Farewells 85

Chapter 16   "Picky, Picky, Picky" 91

Chapter 17   Year-End Appraisals 97

Chapter 18   Stressed Out 103

Chapter 19   Train For Life 109

Chapter 20   Quarantine 115

Chapter 21 Holiday Frenzy 121

Chapter 22 Taking Stock 129

Chapter 23 Fit Pharisee 135

Chapter 24 "No Excuses" Redux 141

About The Author 147

PREFACE

When it comes to physical education, I've always considered myself a slow learner. Not too long ago, I hired someone to teach me how to jump rope. Not that I didn't jump rope; I just knew I wasn't doing it right. It took about three sessions before my deficiency was successfully addressed. Finally, I was able to land on both feet at the same time, instead of kind of skipping in place—a humiliating deficiency that had plagued me for decades.

As a youngster, I could usually be counted on to be among the last of my classmates to be picked for the softball team. The "why" is fairly simple: the only time I would actually hit the ball with a bat was to foul it off my head or jaw. I was marginally better at kickball offense, but only because it required less coordination.

Today, I would probably be told that I was "variously" or "differently" challenged. I also know now that with time and the right kind of guidance, I could have overcome just about any of the physical obstacles I experienced as a child. But what I needed then was not available, at least to me, namely, caring tutelage from teachers/trainers attuned to my specific needs.

This memoir recounts my experiences over the past six years working with two personal trainers, Austin Rowe and Pete Goulet. But in order to put this narrative in context, I think I should spend some time writing about my younger self. As a boomer, there's a lot to cover, but I'll try to do it succinctly.

Like most of my generation, I spent a good deal of time in my twenties and thirties working out at the gym. For me, that meant Payne Whitney at Yale University, a Valhalla of gymnasiums. It was there that I took grueling circuit-training classes with the legendary Delaney Kiphuth and only slightly less rigorous instruction from the jolly Herb Hennessy. Herb's regimen for exercising was playing music that he had recorded on open reel tapes. I found the Venusberg music from Richard Wagner's opera *Tannhäuser* the most invigorating. I'm sure it produced my highest adrenaline levels.

Circuit training may be the most challenging exercise I've ever experienced. Basically, it consists of two rounds of about a half-dozen activities, most of which I've forgotten. Still, two stand out. The first is stepping up and down on a bench for five minutes—twice! If you think that's easy, I invite you to try it. But please consider bandaging your shins before beginning.

The second is medicine ball throwing with/at a partner. For some reason I would invariably be teamed with a bearded brute who clearly did not like me. He lusted for blood when he threw the ball at me. I may have asked him once to lessen the velocity, but that only incited him to throw harder. To this day, he remains my model for how not to partner with someone at the gym.

By the time I reached my thirties, I had moved to Boston, where I worked out briefly in classes given at a grungy loft in the up-and-coming South End. The lack of showers was a definite downer, and I quickly lost interest in returning. Around that time, the spiffy Metropolitan Health Club opened closer to my home, and I signed up—and remained an active member for about a half-dozen years.

Almost all of my activity at that time was unsupervised. Weightlifting was all the fashion then, and it produced some amazingly freakish results—like the guy with a huge chest who strutted around on two spindly, toothpick legs. Or the fleshy mesomorph with Rubenesque biceps—truly freakish. Like them, I did not work out with a personal trainer, and the results definitely showed. There was one occasion when I tore something around my tailbone while bench pressing. I soldiered on, oblivious to the damage I was doing. A trainer would probably have cautioned me to ease up, or might have prevented the injury in the first place. Though truth to tell, trainers back then were more boosters than anything else.

Here, my experience probably follows that of many of you. Working out is pretty easy in your twenties and early thirties.

But then, family and job responsibilities start to accumulate, and your commitment to getting to a gym on a regular basis takes a backseat to these obligations. In my case, I dropped my gym membership around the time I turned forty and wouldn't return until six weeks shy of my sixty-seventh birthday. Those were lost years and I knew that in retirement, I would want to go back to a gym. What I didn't know was that I would commit to working out with a personal trainer.

Joining Equinox Sports Club Boston entitled me to one free session of Pilates and one consultation/workout with a personal trainer. I'm sure Pilates is wonderful for many, but it just wasn't my cup of tea. But training intrigued me since it finally opened the possibility of receiving the kind of personal supervision that I craved but never got in childhood. The demons of fouling softballs off my head would finally be exorcised!

Training for Life is not a how-to manual. I've looked at exercise-for-seniors books and frankly, I don't find them especially helpful because they precisely lack the attention to personal detail that training offers.

Training for Life is personal. It may be helpful to you, I hope so. I also hope it inspires readers to experience working out regularly with someone who knows what he or she is doing. It has made all the difference in my life. It has provided a regular routine to my weekly schedule, it incites self-discipline, it has provided me with two new friends. Oh, and by the way, it has resulted in a thirty-pound weight reduction. I'm forever grateful to my first trainer for dubbing me Benjamin Button, the Brad Pitt character who grows younger with age.

There are two voices in this tale besides my own, and they of course belong to the two trainers, Austin and Pete, who have been part of my journey over the past six years. I hope I do them justice, but any failings or shortcomings herein are squarely mine alone. I owe them my current health and well-being, and for that, I will be forever grateful.

Chapter One

NO EXCUSES

I remember my first session with Austin in 2017. I had retired about two weeks prior and felt it might be worthwhile to work one-on-one with a trainer. So in September I signed up for my free session with a trainer who turned out to be Austin. I had no say in the matter, since Equinox randomly assigned me to him. Not that it mattered; I didn't know one trainer from another.

That first morning, Austin had me carry some dumbbells around; he had me do various balancing acts, and we finished with a ride on a stationary bicycle-on-steroids called the Airdyne. The last experience confirmed just how out of shape I had become without realizing it. My weight had ballooned to 173 pounds. Just five years before, it had been 148. Weight gain can be so insidious. Like getting out of shape, I wasn't especially aware of putting on the extra pounds. Or maybe I was in denial—hard to say.

Riding the Airdyne was a cardio challenge. Today, it would be a piece of cake—oops, forget that image! But in 2017, it really put me to the test. I was definitely out of breath when the hour session ended. But then, as I was walking home, something dramatic happened. I felt euphoric. I guessed that those much-ballyhooed endorphins—in my case chronically dormant—had actually awoken. And right then and there, I decided to sign up for two sessions per week. A month later, the twice-weekly sessions became three.

I look back now and understand that those early sessions were tests or, more precisely, tests of my limits. Cardio, balance, endurance, flexibility, strength—all were being pushed to see just how far I could go. There was even a diagnostic instrument that took my weight and height, told me how fat I was, and spat out a whole host of metrics that I never knew existed. It even issued a report on paper, but I could barely read the results since the Equinox printer was chronically low on ink.

By Thanksgiving, a friend commented that my face looked thinner. I thought that was kind of funny, since I never especially attached weight loss to the head! But by Christmas, the loss was pretty much visible all over. I recall a neighbor seeing me and calling me skinny, which I did not necessarily take as a compliment.

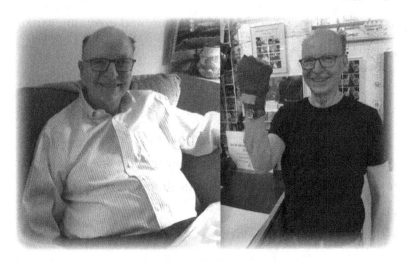

October 2017 versus February 2018

As everyone knows, losing weight and keeping weight off are two distinctly different ballgames, and over the past six years, my weight has fluctuated between 143 and 158. Still, that's significantly under my peak of 173. But it does require work and discipline. An acquaintance of mine once wrote a book about dieting, the essence of which can be summarized as follows: lose weight by eating less and/or exercising more. I'm afraid he was absolutely right, and I work hard at keeping it off every single day.

Which begs the question, why? Why exercise? Why eat less? They don't guarantee that you'll live one day longer. But I think that that defeatist attitude misses the point. Exercise and weighing less are accomplishments that make me feel better and look better. As one of my friends habitually points out, that's because of my narcissism. Maybe, but I also see the wisdom of staying as healthy as possible in one's so-called golden years, and exercising with a personal trainer is a mighty tool for attaining that goal.

—⟋⟍—

In six years of training, I never felt that Austin or Pete have pushed me into a danger zone. Yes, they would sometimes ask me to do something I couldn't do. But in almost every such instance, persistence has paid off.

Here's an example from 2017: envision jumping on wooden boxes from a stationary position. I think the box was twenty inches high, but it could easily have been Mount Everest. Every time Austin said "one, two, three, JUMP," I choked. It was embarrassing and it conjured up the nasty softballs I used to foul off my head.

At first, I didn't know what to do. I intuited that the impediment to jumping was more mental than physical. But that didn't help me to remove the mental block. So I decided to sneak into the weight room when no one was around. I must have gone there six or seven times over two weeks. My strategy was to get a running jump, and then reduce the length of the run each successive time. Sure enough, I jumped successfully from the get go. But just as with jump rope, I was jumping off one foot, not two.

Returning to Austin, I just knew that I would have to psych myself into doing this. And somehow, after several entreaties, I jumped! It was a successful jump and a successful landing, thank goodness. Austin captured the moment on his iPhone and you can still observe the magic moment on my Facebook page.

—⁂—

Young or old, you really can't gain strength if your mobility is impaired. And in those early sessions, we wisely worked on making sure my joints were in working order. Warmups consisted of rotations from the neck down to the ankles, forward and backward, clockwise and counterclockwise. There were two weak points, shoulders and toes. Both had given me problems in the past. I'm one of a rare set of folks who has managed to get *adhesive capsulitis* or "frozen shoulder" in both shoulders. And my right big toe was a special problem—still is today.

I think Austin also suspected that my ankle mobility wasn't quite what it should be because he suggested I buy a cool pair of blue Nordic Lifting shoes that allowed me to get deeper into squats while keeping my spine in what trainers call a neutral position. It didn't hurt that I thought I looked sexier wearing them—or maybe it was the shoes that were sexy, not me. Still, they gave me some added height and confidence, like a short Italian tenor on lifts!

The moral of the tale is that you never know which incentives will nurture your interest and commitment to working out. If it's a pair of blue shoes—I now have two pairs—then go for it. Conversely, don't let temporary "failures" like not jumping on a box get you down. And most important, don't let excuses cripple you! When all is said and done, keep to your plan. I guarantee, you will not regret it!

Chapter Two

TRUE BELIEVER

Anyone who's had a Born Again moment knows what I felt like by the end of 2017. I was a borderline fanatic. On Mondays I was taking boxing classes. Wednesdays were reserved for yoga and Saturdays were tagged for lap swimming. The rest of the week was allotted to Austin, except for the Lord's Day and my day of rest.

Predictably, boxing raised the most howls. "David Lapin, I don't at all see you as a boxer. You've lost your marbles." "You're too old to be doing this. You push yourself too hard." Well fine, thanks for the positivity. The only thing that finally floored me was the shutdown of all class activities during the 2020 pandemic. I haven't gone back to either yoga or boxing, and today, at seventy-two, I figure my boxing days are probably over. But if that's the case, it's because of limits I set for myself. Only you and your trainer can be the judge of how far you can push yourself in any pursuit.

My first boxing class at Equinox was oversubscribed, but Austin spoke to the instructor and miraculously got me in. There may have been one other person my age, which was unsurprising. What was surprising to me was that there were more women than men. And most of them were qualified to land a punch on me before I could say ouch. So much for gender stereotypes.

I quickly learned the basic moves against a punching bag (jab, cross, hook, upper cut), but what really sticks out in my mind today is how much boxing is about legwork. "I dance under those lights" said Mohammed Ali, and now I know what The Greatest One was talking about. We did a lot of running and legwork in class, but I have to say, I never completely got the feeling that I was dancing—"leaden on his feet" is probably the more apt image.

Punching was something else. I always liked punching. My father wasn't averse to occasionally punching someone and I guess I inherited that gene. But landing punches precisely is an art and there I confess I came up short. On one occasion when we were paired with sparring partners, I accidentally landed a punch on my partner's cheekbone. That was a definite no-no since I was supposed to be aiming only for his hand pads. Fortunately, he was gracious about my faux pas and didn't opt to reciprocate.

In the winter of 2018, I left Equinox and Austin for a month to go to South Beach in Miami Beach, or SoBe, as it is commonly abbreviated. The prior winter I had vacationed in Fort Lauderdale and took a day trip to visit friends in South Beach. I was instantly taken by the vibes—both cosmopolitan and Latino—and immediately decided to return the following year. A friend and I leased a two-bedroom apartment at the Decoplage at the corner of Collins Avenue and Lincoln Road, very touristy but oh so nice.

Seeking something akin to the physical regimen I had tailored for myself in Boston, I joined the fabled South Beach Boxing Gym in Miami Beach. It was there that I stepped into a ring for the first time. And let me tell you, I was damn nervous, not about fighting, but just figuring out how to get through the ropes without killing myself. I consider my adult self to be fairly well coordinated, but doing something physical for the first time inevitably shifts me into high anxiety mode. Somehow I vaulted in but then my nerves focused obsessively on how I was going to get out!

Mind you, this is all before actual sparring. My wizened instructor intimidated me intellectually when he feigned punching me in the face and said "What do you do?" "How the hell should I know?" went through my mind, and then, "Just kill me and get it over." He asked me again. Nothing. A third time. By then, I was dripping in ignominy, so he finally took pity on me and said the magic words, "YOU DUCK." "Oh," I eloquently replied, like a James Joyce character experiencing an epiphany.

Once past that awkward moment, I actually enjoyed my time

at South Beach Boxing and re-upped in 2019 and 2020 before Covid put an end to my boxing career. Still, it was time well spent and I now consider this experience one of the signal achievements of my sixties.

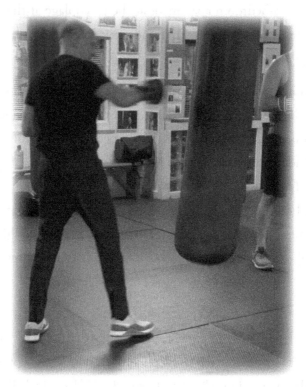

South Beach Boxing

It may sound strange but for me, yoga is harder than boxing. I have never found meditation easy and trying to focus on nothing but breathing can be excruciating business. Even simple poses could elude me when accompanied by meditation or relaxation.

Yoga is a total mind- body workout and it was the focus on the mind that gave me the most trouble.

I recall that the yoga classes at Equinox were graded as something like beginning to advanced, gentle to intense. I tried out all of them, but ultimately found myself most attracted to the gentle approach, reasoning that I got more than enough intensity from boxing. My instructor was a formidable woman who would begin each session with a reading, always from the same book whose title now escapes me. It could have been called Introduction to Generalized Spirituality, which was fine.

I found it curious that during each session she would ask us if we were pregnant or thought that we might be pregnant. This seemed rather odd since aside from the few men, all the women appeared to be between fifty and eighty-five. But somehow, it was endearing and I would look forward each week to hearing that mantra repeated.

I'm not good at describing poses and you can probably get better information from yoga manuals. But I will recommend one pose in particular because, strange as it may seem, it involves the tongue. It's a balancing act. Gently raise your right foot while bending your leg and bringing your foot to the inner side of your left knee. Afterwards, do the same with your left foot. Try keeping this pose for at least thirty seconds. If you can't make it to thirty, try again while pressing your tongue against the hard palate in your mouth. It works, though I never figured out why. Keep pressing and you'll be passing sixty seconds before you know it. Namaste!

Chapter Three

PROPRIOCEPTION

2018 was a year of self-discovery as Austin led me through new routines while I also reacquainted myself with old ones. With the loss of twenty-plus pounds, I was definitely feeling more agile and flexible. I was able to do dead lifts fairly easily because my hip mobility was unimpaired. And since I had no problem with rotating and twisting, I returned to lateral tossing of the medicine ball, where Austin proved to be a far more supportive partner than my Yale nemesis from forty years prior.

I considered these renewals a blessing. I am fortunate that I didn't experience the balance problems that afflict many people of my age. My core strength for everyday activities was reasonably decent. And while I have had chronic back problems and inflammatory disorders, they didn't interfere with my sessions. Austin had a keen sense of my abilities, but he also gave me the confidence to test and expand the perimeters of my comfort zone.

The Equinox environment also proved to be conducive. I remember my first trip there. As I was guided through its two floors, I told the sales associate that I was lost. And indeed, it took a week or two for me to get my bearings. In one concession to my age, I kept my eyeglasses on while working out, not because I needed them to exercise, but because I wouldn't otherwise be able to see the numbers on the locker door where I had left my civvies.

At first, I was like a child opening gifts on Christmas. There were so many new "toys" to play with. But for all the newfangled machines and equipment, I found two old standbys to be the most entertaining. One was a pair of large and long ropes, which Austin would have me pound into the floor, both simultaneously and in oscillating fashion. Good fun but also good exercise. The other was a weighted sled. I was directed either to pull or push the sled along a forty or fifty-foot course of AstroTurf. This I did not find at all easy. But it became a lot more fun when Austin decided to stand on the sled, thereby providing the added weight that I had to push or pull. "Rowe (Austin's surname), Rowe, Rowe your boat, gently down the stream" I would sing—thereby proving that if I could still sing, I probably wasn't carrying enough weight.

I don't recall today whether Austin emphasized pull movements over push. It would make sense, however, if he had since most seniors including me have developed a hunched posture and a flexed spine. What I do remember is his ability to improvise and "make do" with whatever was available—all within the longer endgame of helping me to achieve sustained results. Some of these could be measured by charting declines in body fat, visceral fat (the nasty stuff around organs), and increases in muscle, bone mass and the like. I was also thrilled to see that the measures revealed a metabolic age of 59, where I remain today. I guess metabolic time can stand still.

All of these activities were fine-tuning my sense of my body in space. The word for that is proprioception, and I now think that that sense of developing one's place and movement in physical space is a critical accomplishment that training can facilitate. It's not a fixed goal; indeed, it might be limitless. I know now that an undeveloped proprioception was probably the cause of my physical limitations as a child. Well, to use a well-worn cliché, better late than never!

A dividend of all this body work meant several trips online to Joseph A. Bank, Paul Frederick, and Amazon for new clothes. My suit size went from 42 to 38, and my neck decreased from 16.5 to 15.5. The latter might even have been lower were it not for my damn turkey neck. Apparently that's one set of muscles that doesn't respond to training! The shirts were usually slim or tapered, but not the jeans. I once tried on a pair of slim jeans at Macys and barely managed to peel them off.

For the suits and dress shirts, I was on my own, but for sneakers and athletic wear, Austin was the boss. I've already told you about the blue Nordic shoes, but he also introduced me to Nike sweats and hoodies—even stylish underwear from Under Armour and Puma. He deemed my ultra wide white sneakers dorky, and very generously gave me two pairs of his own more stylish shoes. Today, I consider them keepsakes of my time with him.

I guess you might conclude that I was an aspiring Eliza Doolittle to Austin Rowe's Professor Henry Higgins. Or better still, the Monster to Dr. Frankenstein. Like doctors, barbers, clergy, and diverse shrinks, you may develop a relationship with a trainer that approximates the psychological phenomenon of transference. I even began seeing him in me, especially with the clothing switches, and on one memorable occasion, I even saw his brain enter my head. I happened to be under the influence of bonged California coffee at the time, but you get the picture. Your relationship with a trainer is intense but you always need to remain respectful of the professional boundaries that define the relationship.

I hope that I also had a meaningful impact on Austin Rowe. How else would he know today who soprano Maria Callas was! We had conversations about religion and politics. He is spiritual and I'm an Episcopalian. He is libertarian and I'm an institutionalist. I'd like to think that some of my brain entered his. He challenged me as no one had in years. We even talked about him teaching me to wakeboard on a lake near his family home in a suburb of Boston. Now, that would have been something. Sad to say, we never got around to it, but it was exhilarating just thinking about it. Sometimes it's good to have goals even when they ultimately remain out of reach.

Chapter Four

STORM CLOUDS

Training does not come cheap, at least not if you want a quality trainer. Equinox offered me various discounts for purchasing sessions in bulk, and I took advantage of them as much as I could. Still, the annual cost for the training alone came to about $9,000 or $10,000. Add to that the monthly membership fees and we're pushing $12,000 for twelve months' work.

That's a lot of money, undeniably. And I fully understand that the figure is well above what many seniors can afford. I definitely stretched my budget to make training work. I also got my certified financial planner's de facto endorsement, as he incorporated the cost into his overall plan for my first years in retirement.

On the upside, all my yoga and boxing classes were free. The use of the lap pool was free; it was the presence of a pool that attracted me to Equinox Sports Club Boston in the first place.

In addition to swimming, I typically would do cardio-exercise days on my own. Austin saw no sense in using treadmills when you can walk or run outdoors—at least until New England weather makes that unbearable but for the hardiest among us. (I do not count myself among the latter.)

My default apparatus was my old friend the Airdyne, supplemented by a rowing machine and the elliptical—a device that kind of mimics cross-country skiing. On some occasions I would use the Airdyne and the rowing machine for spurts of high-intensity workouts. On other days I would use them at steady paces for typically thirty minutes. Only after many months would I use the StairMaster, a machine for climbing steps. I had an irrational fear of falling off of it, so once again, I needed to confront my psychological demons before I could incorporate it into my regular routine. And sure enough, I almost did fall off it on my first dismount. Today, I use the StairMaster every week, which is probably wise since I live in an apartment thirty-one floors above Boston harbor. You never know when the elevators might quit!

Equinox incentivized its trainers to reach certain thresholds above which they earned pay bonuses. That made sense to me so when Austin was approaching one of those levels, I might add a session or two to help him over the top. As a new trainer (he had only started at Equinox a few months before I met him), he was receiving their base level of compensation. But during the course of the year, he was promoted, which seemed well deserved and a good thing until I discovered that Equinox required his clients to pay for the increase. That did not seem right at all. Moreover, it defied the laws of economics since folks will always be tempted to move to trainers who cost less. In my professional career, I headed a music school in Boston, and we always insisted on flat tuition rates for students, regardless of what different teachers were paid.

I paid for the increases—there were more than one—because I liked working with Austin a lot and because I was making so much progress. But I also knew that he had lost some clients due to the promotions so his overall salary effectively remained unchanged. This hardly seemed a great way to promote client or trainer loyalty, and I began to hear grumblings from others about this pay-more-for-more-experienced-trainers policy.

As much as I hated the idea, the handwriting was on the wall. Sooner or later (and probably sooner), Austin would leave Equinox. I was really torn about this prospect. On one hand, I dreaded losing him as a trainer and as a friend. We had grown close over the year and I really valued our work together. On the other hand, I knew that his dream was to open his own gym at some point. We began to have conversations about where and when this might happen. At the time, I thought he was too inexperienced and too young at twenty-two to take on such a high-risk endeavor. There were so many unknowns. Where would this take place? Downtown Boston commercial real estate prices were incredibly high in 2018—remember this was the pre-pandemic era. I offered to make a few phone calls to real estate agents about possible locations. The response that I got was fairly uniform: landlords with available venues were usually looking for banks as prospective tenants since they were most likely to afford the sky-high rental rates.

Suburban Boston was an option. But that had scant appeal for me since I don't like driving and wasn't about to shuffle off to a mall by commuter train for training sessions no matter how high my regard for Austin's training skills. The more I thought about it, the more absurd the idea of one person launching a gym seemed.

But then something happened that changed the picture. My boxing instructor was headed to Denver with his wife who was starting a graduate program in the Mile High City. He and Austin began talking and slowly they hatched the idea of opening something together. I thought this prospect made eminent sense. Two principals were better than one to my mind. And Austin's youth would be offset by an older partner with more experience under his belt.

By early summer, a business plan had been drafted and what had begun as conjecture now looked closer to reality. As you can imagine, I still had mixed feelings. I knew that even with two persons committed to the plan, a gym remained a risky enterprise. I think I read once that most small businesses fail after about four or five years, and I certainly was concerned for Austin that this fate might befall him. But basically I was upset over losing my trainer. We had accomplished so much in such a short period. And who would I get to replace him? It was sheer luck that Equinox assigned Austin to me. Why should I presume that I would get lucky a second time!

In August, I departed Boston for my annual pilgrimage to Cape Cod. I had an energetic week, bicycling and walking to the lighthouse on the breakwater rocks at Provincetown Bay. My physical strength, balance and endurance far exceeded where they had been a year ago. But throughout the week, I kept returning to the unpleasant fact that I was about to lose the person who had made all my gains possible.

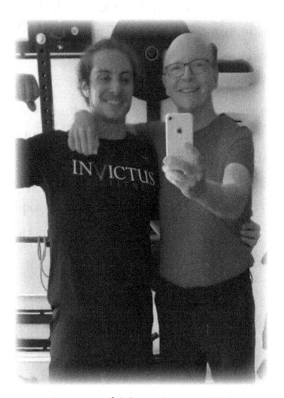

Austin and Me in August 2018

Chapter Five

TRANSITION

A ugust 17 proved bittersweet. In the evening I took Austin out for a farewell dinner at Fleming's Steakhouse in the cozy Bay Village neighborhood of Boston where I had lived since 1980. He had a hamburger as evidenced by the photo I took of him. I can't remember what I had except for a martini. If I had become a training zealot, it didn't impact my consumption of spirits and wine. I don't remember if Fleming's had Plymouth gin, but if they did, that's what I had. Shaken and with olives. I really don't care if shaking bruises the gin. Life can be tough sometimes.

Earlier that day we had worked out at a private studio on Washington Street in downtown Boston not too far from Equinox in a building that had once been exclusively a jewelers exchange. Austin had already given Equinox notice, so our final workouts occurred in that space. Of course it was much smaller than Equinox, but since we were the only ones using it, it proved to be fine.

Our final session involved resistance work with bands around the legs. There were two main activities. One involved placing small, thickish bands around the knees and walking sideways back and forth in a crouching pose, butt out. The second utilized longer and narrower bands tied around a pole on one end and around one of my ankles on the other. We did various repetitions, but basically the idea was to move the tied leg up from the hip toward the ceiling to approximately a forty-five degree angle. Again, the motion was sideways, not forward and back. (I also now visualize Austin with bands around his legs, so he must have been demonstrating the motions to me before I did them.)

And with that, our last session ended. I looked great but felt terrible. A year with Austin Rowe had transformed me from an overweight sexagenarian to a physical specimen as fit as I had been since my thirties, if not younger. Austin was the one who dubbed me Benjamin Button and I was totally flattered by the comparison.

The next morning, I helped Austin and his girlfriend pack his car, and when I say pack, I mean it. The last thing in was a kettlebell, which he couldn't resist using before tossing it into what remained of the trunk space.

"Bye" they both yelled several times as they drove off waving at me. Their new adventure had begun. And, as it turns out, so had mine.

In my last weeks at Equinox with Austin, I began diverting my attention from him and observed other trainers working. I had no interest collaborating with peacocks on steroids, so that eliminated a few of them. There were a couple of women trainers who seemed plausible, but none was clearly superior, at least as I called it. After a time, and with Austin's blessings, my attention focused on a strapping six-foot two-inch guy who always seemed to have a cheery disposition. Austin made the first move and introduced me to Pete Goulet. The handover was more extended than that—Austin and Pete spent some time going over what I had been doing and what my strengths and limitations were—but basically, that was that.

Well, not quite. I had only worked with two trainers: Austin and the capable gentleman who remedied my jump rope pathology in three sessions. I needed to test this new candidate and he needed to test me. I can't tell you how to pick a trainer—the process is so subjective—but it may be helpful to think of it as akin to choosing a dentist. Maybe we boomers would have referred in the day to the Yellow Pages, remember them? Or more likely, we'd get a reference from a friend or colleague. Either way, you're basically going in blind at your first encounter. But after that initial appointment, you usually know whether you want to trust the dentist with your mouth and teeth. I think it's much the same thing with personal trainers.

At first, I didn't observe much difference between Pete and Austin. That probably eased the handover for me, and it was only with time that I discerned how very different they are, both personally and professionally. Trainers have to project enthusiasm for their work with you. If their minds wander off more than occasionally, you probably want to move on. I've seen trainers on their iPhones and Androids during a session. Full stop, red light. Neither Austin nor Pete ever looked at their phones during a session with me.

Pete immediately made me feel comfortable. I felt like he supported me. Perhaps most important, as with Austin, he projected confidence in my ability to reach for new goals. That, in turn, only added to my commitment. We were *simpático* and definitely off to a good start.

I recently told Pete that he was the only trainer who Austin recommended to me. This is absolutely true and I highly valued that recommendation, given the source. Pete is just a few years older than Austin. They are both products of excellent undergraduate education at the University of Massachusetts at Amherst. Austin originally matriculated at George Mason University where he was on the swim team, but a concussion put an end to that nascent career. Pete and Austin overlapped for a couple of years at Amherst, but I don't think they interacted much until they both wound up as colleagues at Equinox.

Pete's ancestry is part Vietnamese, part Chinese, and part Parisian French via Canada—hence his surname, Goulet. Of course, I couldn't help asking whether he had ever heard of the singer Robert Goulet and, of course, he had. It was as dumb a question as people asking me if I know that my last name Lapin means rabbit in French. Anyway, the question and the answer had broken the ice, and I felt reasonably certain that Messieurs Goulet and Lapin would make a good match. And five years later, we're still at it!

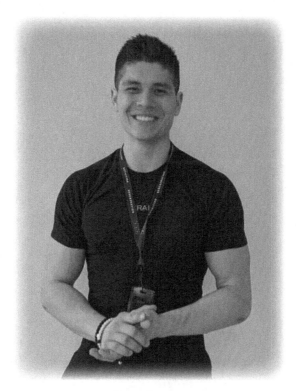

Pete Goulet

Chapter Six

"CAT, COW"

Throughout 2018 and 2019, I traveled frequently, not just in the USA, but to Brazil, Uruguay, Greece, Eswatini aka Swaziland, and South Africa—my first time in each of these countries. All of the journeys were rewarding, but my trip throughout South Africa was extra special for me, as we moved from Pretoria to Kruger National Park, Durban, Capetown and many places in between via the ultra-luxurious Rovos Rail—the "Pride of Africa." I could not have known then how quickly the world would change by March 2020, as almost all international travel was upended. I had hopes that year and the next of visiting Spain and India, but two attempted trips to Spain and one to India were aborted by the virus or "the plague," as an acquaintance insisted on calling it.

Personal training served me in good stead on these adventures. My balance was superior on the highly slippery approach to the Acropolis in Athens. (Too many tourists' footsteps have left the stone almost frictionless.) Climbing to the art deco statue of Christ the Redeemer in Rio de Janeiro posed no problems. And crawling on all fours through a long subterranean cavern in Johannesburg may have stressed me mentally—incipient claustrophobia—but hardly left me breathless. I was a wildebeest in action!

On these sojourns I learned that it's okay to stop training for a while. And on each return, however physically tired I was from the trip itself, I felt spiritually renewed, mentally refreshed, and eager to take on the new challenges that Pete had in store for me.

—ɷ—

The transition from Austin to Pete was made smooth in part because I had returned to the familiar environment of Equinox Sports Club Boston. We settled on two weekly sessions, and in five years, we've rarely deviated from that regimen. I continued my weekly yoga classes, but the loss of my boxing instructor to Denver made my attendance in those classes less frequent, as I did not particularly like his ultra-high energy and noisy successor.

One reform that Pete introduced me to immediately was what he calls "cat, cow." The phrase refers generally to gentle alterations while on one's hands and knees that flex the torso and bring flexibility to the spine. But Pete extended the meaning for me to mindfulness about one's back and spine, especially when bending. For most of my life, I would bend over like a two-legged cat, placing unnecessary strain on my spine and aggravating my all-too-chronic back problems. I think I must have heard him yell "Cow!" at every session for at least a year, most often when doing deadlifts or relearning how to pick up heavy kettlebells and dumbbells. Over time, I would correct myself without his admonishments, though even now I will slip every so often as "Cow!" rings in my ears once again.

As we got to know each other better, we would share our thoughts and observations about other gym regulars. There was a grim fellow who never cracked a smile or said hello. It turns out he had once been an undertaker. There was the language scholar who spent as much time listening to baroque opera on his iPhone and AirPods as he did exercising. And then there were two over-muscled capons who pretty much disdained everyone and kept to themselves in a pact of mutual self-worship. It turned out that both Austin and Pete shared a dislike of them.

My favorite character was a slight guy whom I would regularly observe in an intense stationary bicycle class. I say intense because I have never seen anyone look more pained and appear nearer to death in a gym. As the expression goes, you'd have to see it to believe it. I'm sure he was actually fine, but you'd never know it from appearances. I described the bicyclist and his agonies on multiple occasions to Pete, who couldn't stop laughing as I recounted each new sighting. Sad to say, Pete never got to witness this tortured specimen in action, but we recall him with fondness to this day.

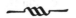

Our first year working out together Pete made continual assessments of my strengths and shortcomings. He had me work for months on the seven movement patterns of something called the Functional Movement Screen (FMS), a tool designed to detect an individual's movement deficits when appropriate stability and mobility are not properly employed. (You can read all about FMS at www.functionalmovement.com.) First up were deep squats. I did not think I did these particularly well, since I was cognizant of the fact that I had squatted much deeper in my twenties and thirties. But the wedged shoes that Austin had recommended for deadlifting definitely improved matters.

Next up was the hurdle step and, no, it's not a dance routine! Hurdle steps challenge step and stride mechanics in a single leg stance. In-line lunges may have been my favorite, though I really can't say why. These were followed by shoulder mobility, active straight-leg raises, trunk stability push-ups, and rotary stability. If all of this sounds technical, it is. I was not even aware at the time that these movement patterns were part of a test, and Pete never shared the results with me. I guess in that regard FMS is like those IQ tests we took in school. At least FMS is a useful diagnostic tool. I'm not sure IQ tests have any value whatsoever.

An exercise from those early sessions that I still do regularly is the plank. I had done planks with Austin as well. My first winter in South Beach, the city was festooned with public trash cans and posters on their sides that read "Plank you for not littering." The illustration on the posters was of a buff guy in plank mode tossing litter into the trash can. I thought that was hilarious.

Doing planks—a core-strengthening exercise roughly akin to an upper push-up position—comes reasonably easy to me and I can hold a plank position for well over a minute. Usually done by balancing between your forearms and toes, your core should assume a feline-like form. Not surprisingly, Pete often yells "Cat!" at me when I'm holding a plank. For most other exercises, if I'm really bad and "doing a cat," he invokes Quasimodo, the hunchback of Notre Dame, and that gets me back to proper cow-form pronto.

Chapter Seven
CONTRASTS

Every few weeks or so, I would get a FaceTime call from Austin, who kept me up to date on his business plan to open a gym. Various neighborhoods in the city were surveyed, and in short order, he and his partner settled on Denver's River North Art District, known affectionately as RiNo. A trendy and artsy area, RiNo had no shortage of industrial buildings suitable for revamping as everything from restaurants to gyms. Faster than I imagined possible, a lease was signed, equipment was purchased, and Apex Human Performance opened for business. It all happened too quickly in retrospect, since multiple problems would afflict Austin and Apex from the start.

The first shoe to drop was the partner. He was missing in action. I found this absolutely astonishing since he was supposedly the seasoned veteran that would bring stability and maturity to the enterprise. So much for that. In any event, his departure left Austin with no one to help run the gym. It also put a large dent in the business plan as boxing classes were a big component of the gym's salability and prospective profitability.

Another problem was the lease. The appeal of the terms was an initial period of six-months free rent. Other than that, the lease was wildly skewed in favor of the landlord, and in his enthusiasm and youth, Austin never had an attorney review the lease before signing it. This omission nearly crippled Apex as disagreements abounded over who was responsible for finishing leasehold improvements, which contractors were to be employed, and how rapidly all the work would be finished. Nonetheless, through Austin's Herculean efforts, Apex quickly gained a steady fan base of paying customers. Despite all the problems, it looked like Apex might buck the trend and survive after all. Austin remained optimistic and I continued to offer a senior's supposed wisdom and encouragement.

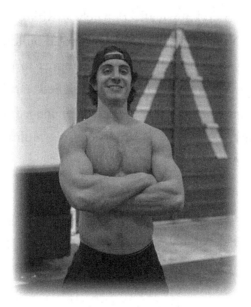

Austin at Apex Human Performance

Meanwhile, Pete and I continued to build on our mutual rapport. The longer I worked with Pete, the more I began to notice differences in my two trainers' training styles and personalities. Austin was open to high-risk behavior, as evidenced not only in starting up Apex, but also in his lifestyle choices. Athletically, he pushed extreme boundaries for himself, whether in mountain biking, wakeboarding, weightlifting, or high-intensity CrossFit exercises and competitions. I expressed concern that any injury he might sustain would jeopardize Apex's viability. These entreaties fell on deaf ears.

Pete tended to be more deliberate and circumspect. While Austin and Pete were both methodical in their training of self and others, Pete only assumed prudent risks. He was the tortoise to Austin's hare. These differences in temperament had implications for their respective approaches to training. In my year with Austin he emphasized strength building and weight training. In contrast, Pete usually has focused our workouts on enhancing flexibility and balance. There is no right or wrong to these different approaches, and both trainers had me do strength and flexibility exercises. But I do believe that Pete's personal strengths and training played more naturally to an older client base, whereas Austin was more suited to working with his peers. Pete has actually told me that he likes working with seniors and relates to their needs. By no coincidence, he has grandparents with whom he is very close. Austin worked superbly with me, but I doubt he considered training seniors his special talent.

Trainers are not Superheroes. They get sick like the rest of us. One day I went to Equinox to find Pete in an atypically low-energy mode. After a few minutes, I could tell that he was severely under the weather. Soreness of throat suggested strep—I had rheumatic fever as a child and could not risk another strep infection—and I urged him to seek treatment. He was in the process of transitioning from his parents' health insurance and wasn't certain his new provider's coverage had kicked in. But as he grew worse as our hour progressed, I insisted that he get immediate medical care. I regularly passed a drop-in clinic on my walk from home to Equinox and I told him I would accompany him there. The walk itself could not have been more than a few hundred steps, but Pete labored to make it. Finally, we arrived, his insurance was accepted, and I left him in the waiting room.

The next day, he texted to tell me that it wasn't strep, it was mono. Antibiotics don't work against viral diseases like mono, but steroidal anti-inflammatories ease the symptoms and in a week or two his symptoms abated. I was glad to have been of assistance. For once, I felt like a trainer who had helped his client. I was also mightily relieved that I had not been exposed again to strep.

As 2018 came to a close, Pete and I exchanged gifts. He gave me a coffee cup with a removable lid, both of which were decorated with music notes—a doff of the cap to my career in music education. I don't recall what I gave Pete, but it was probably bourbon and cash since I'm not especially creative at gift giving. As I look back today at 2018, I consider myself doubly fortunate to have worked with two trainers who contributed to my physical rejuvenation. When I retired in 2017, I committed to engaging in one activity per day. Equinox and my trainers were critical contributors in helping me realize that goal.

Folks often make plans for their post-retirement years. I have a close friend who was going to take conversational Spanish classes. He was going to make audio books from novels for the blind. He also was going to work out. None has been realized. (To be fair, he occasionally goes to the gym.) I'm not sure why I pursue my goals and others don't realize theirs. It certainly affords me no moral superiority, though some suspect that's my real endgame. If anything, I think my active lifestyle in retirement has taken shape out of my fear of doing nothing. Voids in time send me into high anxiety mode. So I have filled the voids with training, music lessons and writing this memoir. I certainly find them far more enjoyable than becoming the proverbial couch potato!

Chapter Eight

FIGHT CLUB

I n mid-January 2019 Equinox Sports Club Boston opened a brand new, dedicated boxing studio. The one where I had punched my unlucky sparring partner in the face was larger, but it was also used for all sorts of non-boxing activities. Equinox invited me to the mini-gala opening and while there was no ribbon cutting, management did get my attention with the wry (rye?) prospect of "Black and Blue cocktails courtesy of KEEL Vodka."

Four "unparalleled personal trainers" walked us through the boxing basics. Two were women, two were men. Somehow I never connected with them personally. The younger woman seemed to hold the most potential, but before I had a chance to work with her, she left Equinox. A year-and-a-half into my tenure at Equinox, I discerned that this turnstile of trainers could be a real problem for me. I even began to speculate whether Pete would also leave.

My commitment to boxing was reaffirmed later in the month when I returned to Florida and South Beach Boxing. Fortunately for me, I encountered the same two instructors with whom I had worked in 2018. (South Beach seemed to do a better job of labor retention than Boston.) Both were also more experienced and had sparred with some of the top-tier prize fighters of the past two decades. I felt privileged to work with them, even as I had to battle my complex over being the oldest boxer in the classes.

South Beach Boxing was hot, and I mean that literally. There was purportedly A/C but it didn't feel like it was on very much. It takes a lot to get me to sweat but beads cascaded off me during my sessions, while my eyes stung with the salt and water that dripped on my lids. The one activity I was forced to curtail was outside running with the rest of the class. My hairless scalp fries in Florida's sun—I don't like hats—and I wasn't about to risk more trips to the dermatologist attempting to keep up with classmates forty years my junior.

The Decoplage building where I stayed had an expansive fitness center, and I availed myself of its equipment. It contained many of the machines and free weights that I used regularly with Pete at Equinox, though I missed his careful eyes and on-point corrections. I got in touch with him after a few weeks had passed, and we scheduled our first virtual training sessions. I tried my best to make them work, but the noise in the gym from canned music and other residents forced me to abort the experiment after two attempts.

I had lots of fun that winter. I watched Michael Tilson Thomas conduct the music of Johann Sebastian Bach and György Ligeti for the New World Symphony in Miami Beach. I thought about going into Miami for *Don Giovanni* or *Madama Butterfly* at the Adrienne Arsht Center, but inertia got the better of me. (I also thought of opera as a kind of cold-weather sport.) I did venture out with three friends to the Everglades and even ate fried alligator for the first time, which—surprise, surprise—tastes like chicken. I attended a cheesy rodeo featuring live alligators. Years before I had gone to a similar sorry event in Fort Lauderdale. At least this time I took some comfort in observing that the poor alligators who performed for us looked a lot healthier if not happier than the old beast that was forced to wrestle with his "caretaker" in that earlier venue.

I also kept in touch with Pete and Austin. Pete would fill me in on happenings around Boston and at Equinox. And Austin kept me up to date on his gym's growing membership. All in all, the month passed quickly. I bade farewell to my instructors at South Beach Boxing, and on February 28, I began the long journey home on Amtrak's *Silver Meteor*.

That train trip "made" my life. I was sitting in a comfy roomette, iPad on my lap, when I suddenly decided to write my autobiography. Two feverish months later, the manuscript was complete, and in September iUniverse published *The Education of Brainiac.* I subtitled it "A New Yorker's Quest for the Good Life in the Hub of the Universe." I assumed that everyone knew that the Hub was Boston, but I overestimated some of my readers' acumen. I'm told I'm often guilty of this charge.

I introduced Austin in chapter forty-nine, lamenting the fact that I hadn't invited him to my retirement gala at the Boston Center for the Arts. Pete became the last new figure in chapter fifty. Pete was good enough to join me that fall at a book-signing party at my old employer, Community Music Center of Boston. He later confided that he felt a little intimidated—all the more reason for appreciating that he showed up to offer his support.

In October I took off for Heathrow on my way to South Africa. I was flying high. Book sales were encouraging. I had scheduled a talk at the Boston Public Library for the winter of 2020. I planned to do a similar event in New York. Of course none of this transpired as the world shut down by the middle of March.

As if launching a book wasn't enough to occupy my time, I also decided to put my home of forty years up for sale. I had high expectations for what I could get; as it turned out, my projections were extravagant. Still, I got a fair price, and packed my worldly belongings for a move in mid-December. I had decided to transition to a high-rise apartment and settled upon one in Boston's West End near hallowed Boston Garden, home to the Celtics and Bruins. The building had a fitness center near the lobby, and that was definitely a plus. And it was roughly equidistant to Equinox as was my old home in Bay Village.

I looked forward to entertaining friends and former colleagues once I returned from Florida in March. I did travel to Manhattan early that month for a performance of *La Traviata* at Lincoln Center. I recall confessing to the patron seated next to me that I had a hunch that this might be our last attendance for some time. And of course, it was. I returned to Boston and bumped on the street into a good friend and gifted musician. He ventured "Let's go for coffee." But by then everything had already closed and we parted ways, unaware that we wouldn't see each other again for almost a year.

The isolation that Covid imposed was overwhelming. I think of myself as reasonably social, but now I was stuck by myself in a new apartment with barely any human contact. I also realized with alarm that my training sessions with Pete were over. Even my building's gym had closed. I was bereft of opportunities to exercise and the wonder is how I got through the next few months without cracking up entirely.

Chapter Nine

WINTER WALKS

With gyms closed and no sense of when they might reopen, I had to make major changes to my exercise game plan. For the first time, I contemplated adding long walks to my weekly regimen. Fortunately, the winter proved relatively mild in temperature and snowfall, so I was able to get out and about fairly often. My favorite routes took me to Charlestown where I would travel first to the U.S.S. Constitution—Old Ironsides—and then head off to the Bunker Hill Monument. Another option was to head towards downtown—a ghostly site almost bereft of humans—and then walk to South Station, finally turning back to Boston Common and the Public Garden.

The longest trip was also the most scenic. I would cross the Charles River into Cambridge, where my first stop was the Museum of Science, whose front lawn featured a masked Tyrannosaurus Rex—gallows humor, Covid style, I surmised. Then I'd walk along the Charles, past the Massachusetts Institute of Technology campus on my right, and circle back home via the Massachusetts Avenue bridge and Back Bay's fabled Esplanade, the scenic backdrop for the Boston Pops' annual Fourth of July performances of the *1812 Overture* and *Stars and Stripes Forever*.

The biggest challenge of these outdoor workouts wasn't the walking. It was timing bathroom visits. With the city shut down, there was absolutely no place along these routes to relieve myself. I even lost it once between South Station and the Common. Once was enough! Henceforth I would be absolutely certain to visit the bathroom before departing, regardless of whether or not Mother Nature was calling at the moment.

—m—

Despite my failure at virtual training with Pete when I was in Florida, we quickly adapted to the new realities and resumed twice-weekly sessions from our respective homes, courtesy of our iPhones and Wi-Fi. The iPhone camera proved amazing. (I was probably using the iPhone 10 at the time.) It seemed to pick up every flaw in my movements. I even came to believe that it was better in some respects than direct observation. It took a while to learn how to position the phone so Pete could follow me. "Angle me up" came to be his latest refrain. But after a few weeks, I became an expert and wasted less time in setups.

Doing training sessions in my living room afforded me the quiet that I required for listening to Pete. That was certainly an advantage over our virtual experiments in Florida. But what was I going to do about my lack of equipment? I still had the foam roller that Austin had left behind, but that was about it. Here, Pete proved to be amazingly inventive. We used books for weights. My sofa was drafted into service for modified pushups and Bulgarian split squats—a version of a single-leg squat where the back leg is elevated on the couch seat. He had me purchase a fifteen-pound, yellow resistance band from Amazon for about eleven dollars. Tying it around door handles and furniture legs, I could do a full range of strength-trainings and stretches, both with my arms and my legs.

He even introduced me to a new core exercise called the Standing Pallof Press. All I needed was a doorknob and my yellow band. I placed one end of the band around the outer knob and closed the door on it. I grabbed the middle of the band and slowly moved it away from my body for a full extension. I then bent my elbows and returned the band to my navel, while avoiding twisting my core in the process. Pete actually filmed me doing a Pallof Press and posted it on his Instagram and Facebook pages where it garnered over three-hundred views in its first week or two online.

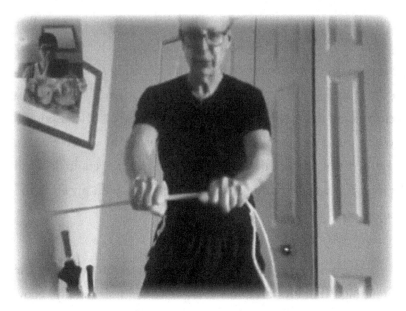

A screenshot of me doing the Pallof Press
Note Pete observing in upper left corner.

In pre-Covid days at Equinox, I had always warmed up prior to my training sessions with various stretching and limbering-up routines. In my living room throughout 2020, these were distilled into three principal drills. I began by lying on my yoga mat parallel to Austin's foam roller. One bent knee stayed on the roller as I would swing my top arm clockwise ten times, and then counterclockwise, all the while watching my hand encircling me, keeping my knee squarely on the roller and my bottom leg parallel to it. These were variants of sideways thoracic rotations, or rotations for short.

I followed the rotations with 90/90 hip stretches. 90/90 refers to your leg placements on the floor, and while they're a tad complicated to describe, you can watch different versions of these on YouTube. All of them, rightly done, promote mobility, deep breathing and a cow-like spinal position.

The third routine was not my favorite so I would save it for last. It is called Spider-Man after you guessed it. Again, there are many variants, but mine involved extending one leg out sideways while keeping the sole of the shoe squarely on the floor. The other leg was bent at the knee as I attempted to squat as deeply as possible, again retaining a Spider-Man spinal position. These were not easy to do properly, but they did pay dividends in stretching my inner thighs especially.

With these out of the way, I then used the roller on either legs or arms, depending on what Pete had in store for me that day. If I felt especially energetic, I would roll everything, as this comprehensive strategy almost certainly yielded the most positive results.

Equinox was big enough and sufficiently well capitalized to withstand the first Covid shutdown. They even sanctioned their trainers' offsite sessions like the ones I had with Pete. This meant a change in policy, but one that enhanced their customers' commitment to remaining Equinox members during the pandemic. "Stay the course" seemed to be the prevailing sentiment.

As I "stayed the course" as best as I could with Pete, my thoughts frequently turned to the perilous circumstances that Austin confronted in Denver. Apex had prospered member-wise, but not yet sufficiently to turn a profit. Meanwhile, leasehold-improvement and other bills were coming due, even as Covid relentlessly tightened its grip on the economy. The miracle is that Austin pulled through that summer with high hopes for better days once the virus passed from the scene. Sad to say, Covid reality would undercut his optimism.

Chapter Ten

SOLITARY CONFINEMENT

My calendar from Friday, March 9, 2020 until the Saturday before Easter on April 12 noted various appointments, including a massage scheduled for the Equinox spa on March 17. All of these were canceled. My first actual social venture during Covid's initial onslaught took place on Easter Sunday, when I walked two-and-half miles to visit a couple for dinner in the South End. Some restaurants had already reopened for takeout—only a few had set up outside seating since it was still too chilly for comfort—and we feasted on a fine lamb dinner, courtesy of the French bistro Monsieur Robert. The logistics of takeout still needed improving, however, as the restaurant first sent over a single portion of beef bourguignon or some variation thereof. After a few frantic calls, our lamb finally arrived with all the accouterments, better late than never. And I got to take home the beef as a bonus.

That evening I returned on the Tremont Street bus. As it arrived, I observed that there were no passengers. It was empty, aside from the driver. I had to enter through the rear door since the entire front of the bus had been cordoned off to protect the driver from catching the virus. The meager upside was that no fare was collected.

By mid-spring my hair was longer than it had been since the seventies—at least that shrinking portion of my head where hair still grew. Finally, the Governor allowed salons and barbershops to reopen and on May 2 I walked again to the South End for my first haircut since February. With mask in place, I waited outside until a minute or two before my appointment, when I was ushered in to be seated in my barber's chair. The haircut proceeded normally except for the mask. I had to remove my mask straps first on one side, then on the other, so my sideburns and temples could be trimmed. I walked back that day for fear of using the subway, which to my mind still posed an unnecessary risk.

My constant support throughout these dreary months was Pete. In one session, Pete's mother spontaneously appeared on camera in their living room. I told her that her son was responsible for helping to maintain my sanity during Covid. I knew then why solitary confinement is such a cruel punishment. I thought of Nelson Mandela and what he had endured. Fortunately, the first phase of Covid isolation was coming to an end, as summer portended a decline in the virus's spread. For me, as with most folks—single or partnered—it couldn't have arrived a day too soon.

By July, gyms were allowed to reopen. Rules on masking and limits to attendance had to be strictly observed. I needed to check in online each time before arriving and attest that I didn't have Covid or was proximate to someone who had it. These seemed like minimal requirements under the circumstances. I was just glad to be back!

Pete had begun wearing masks before the shutdown. I had not, at least while working out, and the new masking strictures proved daunting for me. First, there was the problem of fogging eyeglasses. I tried applying an anti-fogging goo, but that just smeared things to a blur. Then there was the challenge of hearing. Like most folks my age (think rock generation), I had already sustained some hearing loss. I compensated for this by following people's lips as they talked to me. I didn't realize how important this stratagem had become until masking robbed me of it. Pete would give me instructions, and I often wouldn't have a clue what he said. It was like someone turned off the subtitles in a foreign-language movie.

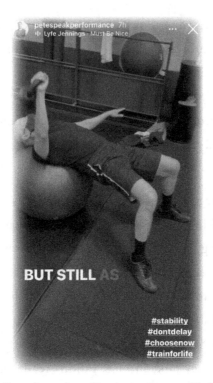

Kettlebell and mask at Equinox Sports Club Boston

Finally, I began cheating. Stretching and mild exercise were mask compatible; Airdyne cycling and full-body exercise were not. Whenever we were alone, I began to pull the mask down below my nose so I could at least breathe more easily. Pete would stand guard to alert me when anyone else came close. I knew that lowering my mask theoretically put Pete at a heightened risk of contracting something from me, but we always tried to maintain the recommended six-feet distance rule—yet another reason why hearing became such a problem.

As had been the case since 1989, I planned on spending the second week of August in Provincetown on Cape Cod. I had already booked my usual two-bedroom apartment overlooking Commercial Street. But then, two shoes dropped. The first was my traveling partner's decision to cancel. Despite all the outdoor activities one can pursue on the Cape, he just felt that the indoor risks remained too high. I thought that those risks were manageable, but I respected his point of view. The second was the final blow. My landlady emailed to say that she needed the apartment for herself and her wife since they had temporarily abandoned their primary residence in Cambridge. Moreover, they didn't feel comfortable having anyone else in the apartment under the circumstances. I had already signed a lease but I wanted to be mindful of her concerns. I also didn't want to do anything to jeopardize my return in 2021. So I emailed back to tell her I completely understood.

Undeterred, I got in touch with the couple with whom I shared Easter dinner to see if they would be interested in joining me for a week. They were game, and due to the numerous cancellations that Covid had provoked, we were able to secure a two-floor apartment with swimming pool privileges. The problem was, when we signed the lease, swimming pools were off-limits. Still, we hoped for the best and happily, the pool opened before our weeklong stay, though we weren't allowed to rearrange lounge chairs on the deck or sit too close to anyone else. I think there were also limits on the number of swimmers that could be in the pool at any one time, but since there were never more than two other guests, we didn't find that restriction odious. We were just glad to see some normalcy return.

Our apartment came with one bicycle, which I very much wanted to use. My plan was to cycle to Race Point via the scenic trails in the Province Lands, as they are called. Then I would return along a different route via Herring Cove Beach. Probably about seven miles into my ten-mile trip, the pedals gave way and divorced from the chain, leaving me effectively immobilized. Fortunately I was only about a mile from Herring Cove, so I walked back to civilization, where one of my comrades and his SUV came to my rescue—sparing me the unwanted exercise of traipsing three more miles back to town with a broken bike in tow.

Chapter Eleven

A DEEP CHILL

The euphoria of the reopening turned out to be short lived. On September 3 my brother died in Winter Park, Florida. Cause of death was listed as "a. squamous cell carcinoma of head and neck" and "b. malignant melanoma." I had been aware of the former. A rare carcinoma formed on his cheek under his left eye and traveled insidiously along a narrow channel toward the brain. Surgical removal was attempted but there was just so far the surgeon could go without risking cognitive impairment. As for the melanoma, that was a surprise to me. I actually doubted whether he had melanoma, thinking that since death from carcinoma is extremely rare, the signing registrar simply added melanoma to make a more convincing declaration.

With my fair skin and genetic predisposition, I have myself had several bouts of skin cancer, so far limited to my scalp. With two surgeries behind me, I felt blessed that, unlike my brother, I've come through them unscathed. I now annually undergo photodynamic therapy, and periodically apply both chemo salves and immune response-enhancing ointments. All of this sometimes make me feel like King Canute holding back the tide.

As much as I like being outside and exercising under the sun, I know my sun days are over. I will only swim outdoors when the sun is down, and outdoor running is strictly verboten— particularly with my aversion towards wearing hats. I'm okay with this. As we get older, if we're lucky, we reconcile ourselves to new limits. If wisdom does come with age, it also deftly helps us to live as gracefully as we can.

—m—

As if our lives were controlled by the Furies in Greek myth, Covid returned with renewed ferocity as summer ebbed and we returned indoors. I have repressed much of the last couple of months of 2020. Oh yes, there was an election. I was still at Equinox on Saturday, November 7, when the race was called four days after Election Day. Honking horns outside the Sports Club gave the results away. Shortly thereafter, state and city governments mandated another round of closings, and I was consigned anew to my living room void.

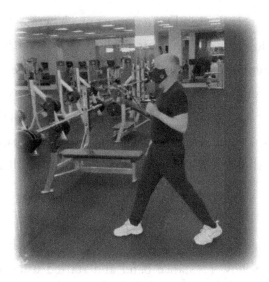

Single arm, high-to-low row in split
stance—at an empty Equinox

Thanksgiving was pretty pathetic. I bought a turkey breast on a quick foray to Whole Foods, and prepared my sides, including the usual cranberries and baked acorn squash. I had also placed a special order for kishka or stuffed derma, a Jewish specialty akin to stuffing made from matzo meal and chicken fat—not especially healthful, but definitely comforting. I had it shipped from Katz's Delicatessen in New York. As for actual human company, there was none. I FaceTimed with a few friends and we ate our respective meals in our brave new virtual world. I guess it was better than nothing, though not by much. Still, I was grateful that we got together at all. Had Covid surfaced before Skype, Zoom and FaceTime, we would have been in a much darker place.

The state of affairs in Denver wasn't much better. Apex wasn't forced to close, but Austin contracted the virus, requiring him to leave the gym and quarantine for two weeks. People often seek out gym memberships in the weeks after Christmas and New Year's, so at least there was hope that an anemic holiday season would turn around in January. But the prospect of subsequent, mandated shutdowns did nothing to help his small business's chances.

I returned to my virtual sessions with Pete. I graduated from my single, yellow resistance band and started using three flat straps in yellow, red and green—each with different resistance levels. These could be used singly or in combinations. As much of a physical fitness buff as I had become, I was relieved that Pete only asked me on rare occasions to deploy all three bands at once. That was tough since combining two proved sufficiently challenging.

In addition to the Pallof presses that I had learned to do with my yellow band, we did a fresh variety of routines, including banded back rows, straight arm pulldowns, and banded chops. For the first, I would thread my straps around a doorknob as if I were doing a Palloff press. After closing the door, I would then engage in rowing motions, bringing the straps back toward my chest. I've seen videos of trainees doing these on one foot. I guess it's possible, but if you're a senior (or even if you're not), your balance has to be fairly strong if you're not going to risk tipping over. Pete never had me do banded back rows on one foot, and I think that was prudent.

Straight arm pulldowns recalled a torturous exercise machine I had used at Equinox with Austin and Pete. With hips at about a thirty or forty five-degree angle, you establish an arc with your arms, bringing them down with elbows locked until your hands align with your hips. Austin had me do these repeatedly and rapidly as intensive cardio assignments, and I did not particularly enjoy being reminded of them in their home reincarnation.

Banded chops are not a cut of meat. For these, I would wrap my straps around a doorknob or the leg of a cabinet and move them with elbows locked across my core from a low to a high angle. The trick here is keeping your core from moving or twisting too much—and also keeping your furniture in place. I didn't want my cabinet traveling with me!

Another routine whose name I don't recall had me lying on the floor on my back with knees bent. On one occasion, I had already wrapped two straps around the leg of my stereo console. I brought my hands over my head until my arms were almost fully extended. But the stereo equipment wasn't heavy enough, and I could palpably feel the console tipping toward me. Fortunately, I released the tension before the console came crashing down on me. There's a reason why we go to gyms to use professional equipment!

Chapter Twelve

WELCOME REBOOTS

New years bring forth optimism—"turning over a new leaf" as the saying goes. And there was real cause for hope in January 2021, as my hometown upstart Moderna competed with the behemoth Pfizer to get a new kind of vaccine to the market—mRNA medicines that identify and instruct specific proteins to prevent or ameliorate certain diseases. The promise was great. But the question remained as to whether or how long it would take to do battle against the coronavirus.

Optimism was also tempered by the sad events of January 6, which I watched unfold live on television. How could this happen in America? Were we no better than the proverbial banana republics? Like so many, I looked on in utter disbelief as I simply couldn't process the images before my eyes. Years ago, I had earned a Ph.D. in political science. As a onetime scholar of American politics and a traditionally proud citizen of the "Good Ol' U.S.A.," I was ashamed and disgusted by the violent turn that that day took.

For a short while thereafter, working out seemed less important. I briefly experienced a mental funk which lifted only when Inauguration Day came and went without further disturbances. We had indeed turned over a new leaf. I also hoped against the odds that we would begin a process of healing and reconciliation.

—◆—

Toward the end of the month, I visited my primary care physician for my annual physical exam, or what Medicare now calls a "wellness visit." (Okay, I know technically they're not the same.) My weight checked in at 155 pounds, four ounces, with clothes on and shoes off. My blood pressure had crept up slightly from the previous year to 144/82 and my pulse was typically high at 90. My temperature was low at 97 degrees—probably due to chronic slight anemia. I don't put much store in the body mass index, but I was gratified nonetheless that mine registered as 22.92–not too shabby for a seventy-year old male. The only red flags she identified were palpitations and APC or atrial premature contractions. My cardiologist had already discussed these conditions with me, so I wasn't surprised to hear about them again. Basically, I was a healthy, fit senior. All my work had paid off and I reported the good news to Pete at our next session.

Throughout the winter we continued to meet virtually. I remained in awe of Pete's capacity to keep our sessions fresh with a balanced repertoire of old and new routines. I wondered how much my sessions resembled those of his other clients. I knew, for instance, that he worked with a senior with Parkinson's. He described how the disease caused its victim's world to grow smaller and smaller. So he would emphasize big movements to try and limit the decreases as much as possible.

My mobility, in contrast, was high for my age, thus Pete could regularly offer me a full palette of large and small movements. Among the latter were Superman poses on my stomach, where I would do banded Y, W and T motions with my arms while my legs hovered off the ground. I found these especially onerous—they didn't at all make me feel like Superman. I candidly expressed my sentiments to Pete, which of course prompted him to have me do them even more frequently. I just thought they brought out the Clark Kent in me.

—⚒—

By the end of February, both Moderna and Pfizer took their vaccines to market in an amazing triumph for American pharmaceutical companies, warp speed, indeed. It all seemed too good to be true, but the real challenge for me was getting a dose into my veins. Even as an ostensibly high-risk senior, I had trouble qualifying for it from my usual providers. I had already decided to return to Florida in March, come hell or high water, and I desperately wanted to have at least one of the two jabs before I left.

As my March 3 departure came ever closer, I grew increasingly anxious. After exhausting all my options at the public website set up for securing appointments, I got a call from a friend who had just booked an appointment through Boston Medical Center, the city's historic leader among hospitals for health equity. The secret for success was abandoning the overloaded website and calling BMC directly. I think that I called on Friday, February 26, and was told that there was an opening on Tuesday, March 2 at 3:45 PM at a community center in the distant Dorchester section of the city. "I'll take it!," I said, mindful of the fact that I would be South Beach-bound at 6 AM the following morning. It didn't even occur to me to speculate whether side effects might prevent me from leaving so soon after my shot.

Getting to Dorchester was an adventure in itself. Public transportation was practically out of the question, though I entertained taking the subway to neighboring Jamaica Plain and praying that I could find a taxi for the rest of the trip. I still hadn't mustered the confidence to return to subways, so I ultimately decided on securing a Lyft or Uber. Even with GPS, the driver found locating the site a challenge. I did get there on time, filled out the requisite forms, and waited my turn. The whole process was reminiscent of voting on Election Day. Finally, I got my jab. I asked whether it was Moderna or Pfizer. I was told it was Moderna, which pleased me no end since I thought for some reason that it probably yielded greater efficacy. I got my COVID-19 Vaccination Card and was told to return for my second dose at 12:10 PM on April 6. By that time I would have gone to and returned from Florida.

Boarding my American Airlines flight the following morning (without side effects), I felt incredibly lucky. Not only had I avoided coming down with Covid. I had also lucked out in getting the vaccine in a timely fashion. I doubt whether it actually helped me fight off the virus on the plane that morning, but I felt better psychologically, and I looked forward to making the most out of my stay at the Hilton Bentley Miami/South Beach.

Chapter Thirteen

RISK/REWARD

Four days after my arrival in South Beach, I met a friend from Boston. I had made reservations at the Red Steakhouse at the southern tip of the city, and we ate outside that evening, in part because of the balmy weather, but also to mitigate risk of contagion. It was still much too cold to indulge in outdoor dining in Boston, so we felt doubly appreciative of the opportunity that the occasion afforded us.

Like most hotels that winter, the Bentley was far from capacity, though I did encounter more fellow guests than I anticipated. Fortunately for me, almost none of them showed an interest in using the hotel's gym, so Pete and I were able to resume our twice-weekly sessions without bothering other guests with my iPhone's speaker. And for once, I could actually hear his instructions since there was no canned music or other background noise.

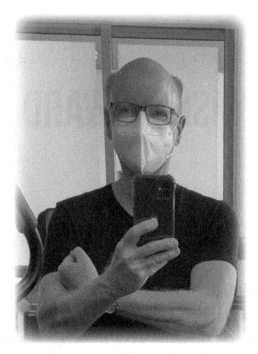

Posing at the Hilton Bentley

The challenge for Pete in training me in venues like the Bentley gym was not knowing ahead of time what kind of equipment was available. I started the hour by scanning the room so he could see what we might use, but decisions on how the session would unfold were pretty much impromptu. Once again, flexibility and creativity became his strengths—and redounded to my benefit. If a gym floor looked like it hadn't seen a mop in a while, he simply had me focus on bench and standing activities. If a Swiss ball or balance ball was present, he'd find a way to work it into our routine. Ditto for kettlebells and dumbbells. And he never seemed irked or frustrated if something went missing. I doubt that one learns these strategies in coursework to become a personal trainer. I think he just came about them naturally.

To add some spice to life (as if anyone needed extra spice in 2021), I decided to transfer after six nights to the Gale South Beach, a Curio Collection hotel also in the Hilton family. This boutique venue is practically in the middle of South Beach, on Collins Avenue near Lincoln Road, close to the Decoplage where I had resided the previous three winters. My room was—to put it politely—cozy. Big spaces were definitely not the Gale's selling points. But there was a splendid rooftop pool, and I took advantage of it several times throughout my stay.

One thing I had noticed at the Bentley and subsequently at the Gale was the lack of masks among guests and hotel workers. Absence of masking was far from universal, but it stood in striking contrast to the situation I had left behind in Massachusetts. Someday, epidemiologists may confirm whether masking really constrained the spread of the virus. My own hunch is that it probably did in northern states, where folks spent more time indoors during colder months. But in Florida, with its outdoor lifestyle, masking probably was less necessary. In any event, I kept mine on for the most part throughout my stay, though not poolside.

Before leaving the Gale, I afforded myself one final scrumptious meal at Forte dei Marmi, a hidden gem of a restaurant on Ocean Drive. I made a mental note to myself to return there, as I deemed it to be one of the superior restaurants in Miami Beach. And with that, I left the city, confirmed in my belief that traveling during Covid was a risk well worth taking.

My trip north was again via Amtrak's *Silver Meteor* in my own private roomette. Federal regulations remained pretty strict at that time and masking was required in all the public spaces on the train. My sleeping-car accommodations afforded me some relaxation, since we weren't mandated to mask in our own rooms unless the attendant was also present. I have always found train travel far more restful for mind and body than taking planes. Sad to say, the train was pretty empty on this occasion. I got to New York on time, met a friend for an hour's layover, and boarded the next northbound Acela for the final leg of my journey to Boston.

The day after my Boston arrival, without skipping a beat, I resumed my training sessions with Pete. I'm not sure exactly when Equinox opened again, but for the next few weeks, we continued our collaboration online.

Like many people, I deferred medical and dental attention in 2020—not that there was much choice in the matter—but I had been scheduled for a once-delayed colonoscopy at the end of the month, and I was loathe to put it off again. I needed to get a Covid-negative result prior to the procedure and I dutifully showed up for my test at Mount Auburn Hospital in Cambridge, which proved negative. I was less lucky with the colonoscopy results as three polyps had to be removed. Fortunately, all were benign. Nonetheless, the doctor recommended that I return in three years, rather than the standard five. I will heed this counsel.

—〰—

By April, restaurants had reopened for both outdoor and inside service, and twelve of us were able to enjoy an Easter dinner reunion at the Harvest restaurant in Harvard Square. Gyms also were allowed to resume business and I finally returned to live sessions with Pete at Equinox.

Prior to the pandemic I had started seeing an Equinox Spa massage therapist whose methods and language were unorthodox, to say the least. English was not the masseur's native tongue, and as a result, he would often have a little difficulty expressing himself. I would have even more trouble discerning what he meant. On one occasion he told me that I had "weak skin, but that's not bad." I told this to Pete, who had recommended the masseur to me in the first place. We laughed at the notion of my weak skin, though neither of us ever figured out just what the heck this meant. At least, it wasn't bad!

Despite the language hurdles, we established a good therapist-client relationship and I was happy to resume my massages on April 21 after a year's absence. It's hard for me to explain how his technique differed from other massage therapists. But it basically came down to a more vigorous manipulation of the body in a multitude of positions, with body parts both on and raised off the table. On one occasion I could have sworn I levitated. It was an amazing moment. Unfortunately for me, he has retired from message therapy, and since I am now spoiled for life, I have yet to find an adequate replacement.

Chapter Fourteen

A LUNCH DATE

Apex Human Performance benefited from the return of springtime to Denver as more folks signed up for monthly memberships. Austin finally found the means to hire a boxing instructor and he remained confident that boxing would enhance both the gym's overall offerings and appeal. A local influencer and fitness buff heavily promoted Apex on social media. And Austin honed his own marketing skills, publicizing in effect both the gym and himself. His personal Instagram account, Austin Rowe Fitness, ultimately attracted over seven-thousand followers. I was mightily impressed not only by this stunning achievement, but also by his overall survival skills in the worst of times.

I had originally intended going out to Denver in 2020, but as that proved impossible, I thought sometime in 2021 might work. But despite traveling to Florida and my own desire for a reunion (not to mention my first anticipated tête-à-tête with Apex mascot Oakley, a pup German shepherd), I remained reluctant to commit to places as far from Boston as Colorado. I felt badly about this—though apparently not sufficiently to move myself off my duff.

We did FaceTime often. I offered what I hoped was reasonable advice, particularly in handling chronically delinquent contractors. Multiple problems abounded largely as the result of the one-sided lease. I even got in touch with a Denver attorney who had been an old high school chum. But the bottom line was always the same no matter who we turned to: the lease was signed, it is what it is, and better luck next time.

—ℳ—

Now in my third year of training with Pete, I had gotten to know a lot about him, as did he about me, of course. I knew that his family came first for him—from his parents to his sister to his grandparents. He told me about the women he was dating and what attracted him to them. He even confided in what he wanted in a life partner. Pete is definitely and emphatically a regular guy.

Pete was also proud of his Asian heritage. As it happens, Equinox Sports Club Boston abuts Chinatown and its many diverse restaurants from all varieties of Chinese cuisine to Vietnamese to Thai and even Asian vegan. He told me that one of his favorite holiday dishes was a rice and gravy concoction that sounded absolutely delicious. One day he mentioned that he'd like to take me out for lunch. It turned out that we had never been physically together outside Equinox, aside from our trip to the health clinic in 2018. I was delighted to accept, and on Wednesday, May 18, we met at noon at New Golden Gate Seafood Restaurant on Beach Street in Chinatown.

I must say that at first it seemed odd sitting opposite him in a restaurant. I was momentarily at a loss for words, but the ice broke fairly quickly as Pete took the lead in ordering food from the menu. Some moments later, I was not disappointed by the plates set before us. Clearly, he had picked dishes that he had previously tasted and enjoyed, and now it was my turn to benefit from his discerning palate.

That day we may have had fish at New Golden Gate Seafood Restaurant, but the dish I especially remember—largely because I took a photograph of it—was a Hainanese chicken and rice combo with stir-fried pea shoots that presented one slight visual problem for me. The chicken appeared undercooked—probably because it had been steamed or poached. But once I overcame that aesthetic blinder, I discovered it tasted fantastic! I even doggie-bagged the leftovers and took them home for a late evening snack. (The photograph shows my chopsticks on the left side of the meal since I am left handed. I learned from a visit to China many years before that this is definitely not considered kosher—to mix ethnicities—in Chinese culture.)

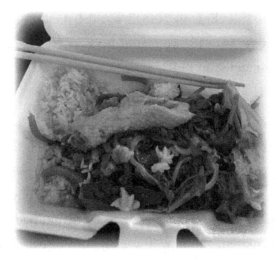

Chicken and rice at New Golden Gate

We ended lunch and walked a few blocks to get coffee at an outdoor cafe on Washington Street. Ever the gentleman, Pete picked up the tab for lunch; I may have paid for the coffee. We said our goodbyes and I walked home, all-the-more mindful of just how fortunate I was to have both Austin and Pete in my life.

That summer, I began experiencing sharp pains in my left foot. Walking became increasingly difficult, and I would have to shift my balance to the right foot to lessen my discomfort. I discussed the problem with Pete and my massage therapist, who spent much of one session trying to address the problem. But nothing seemed to work, as my hobbling increased almost by the day.

Finally, in July, I went to visit my nurse practitioner, who referred me to a podiatrist. As a child with ingrown toenails, I had once waited in a podiatrist's office for hours, so it was with some trepidation that I made the appointment. It didn't help that his office was way out in western Cambridge. Nonetheless, I took a train and a bus—I was over my apprehension about subways by then—and dutifully appeared on August 16 for my 9 AM appointment.

The crowded waiting room did nothing to allay my anxiety. But I didn't have to wait hours before being ushered into two examination rooms, one to see the doctor and the other to take an x-ray of my foot. Finally, the podiatrist gave me his diagnosis. I had "Covid foot," a malady that he was treating at near-epidemic levels. People had gone around their homes for a year without shoes or in slippers and flip-flops. When they returned to wearing shoes, the feet rebelled. In my case, the center of gravity in the left foot had shifted from the big toe to the second and third toes—producing the pain I was experiencing. The short-term solution was a shot of cortisone. The long-term solution was to train the foot to bear weight where it properly belonged on the ball of the foot and the big toe. He recommended ABEO orthotic insoles for my shoes, as well as Birkenstocks for casual wear. Later that day, I went to Macy's for the Birkenstocks and ordered my insoles online.

In finishing up with me, the doctor commented only somewhat in jest that Covid had become a profit leader for him—not unlike the uptick in business that home improvement centers had enjoyed. We laughed and I departed. On my way home, I chuckled over the fact that I finally had to count myself as a collateral victim of the virus—if in a manner that was wholly surreal and unexpected.

Chapter Fifteen

FAREWELLS

May 2021 marked Pete's departure from Equinox. The handwriting had been on the wall for a while. He was making more money working with his own private clients, and his supervisor at Equinox wanted him to commit to more time working for them. It just made no economic sense for Pete and after back-and-forth offers and counteroffers, both parties agreed to an amicable divorce. Pete was on his own, and he branded his new enterprise Prime Core Fitness.

I continued to see Pete outside Equinox, and for the time being I also remained a member of the Club. I owed the company a lot: two excellent trainers, my introduction to boxing and yoga, not to mention the regular use of a superb gym facility and swimming pool. My overall experience could not have been better. And yet, I had a decent fitness center in my own apartment building, which I began using more frequently. By year's end, I decided to let my Equinox membership lapse. I had four wonderful years with them, but I had already intuited that it was time to move on.

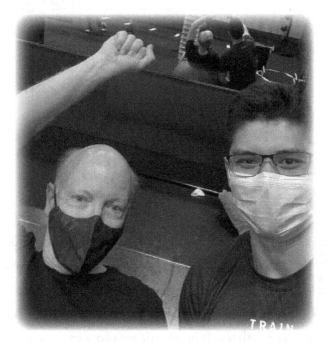

Our last day together at Equinox

Summer 2021 proceeded far more normally than the one the year before. Pete rejoined the rest of his family for their annual reunion at a campground in Dennis Port on Cape Cod. Austin hiked and mountain biked in Colorado's and Arizona's national parks. And I returned to my old apartment in Provincetown, the one that was off limits in 2020. "Status quo ante" sounded like a happy refrain—at least for me. Of course, that meant overlooking the inconvenient fact that by September 18, 2021, the World Health Organization recorded over four and a half million deaths worldwide from the coronavirus. On September 20, The Boston

Globe reported that Covid-19 deaths in the United States had exceeded those caused in 1918 by the influenza epidemic.

I knew that I was repressing many of the tragic events that surrounded me. Up till then, I had not lost any close friends or colleagues to the virus. That afforded me some consolation. And there were happy events to celebrate, including the birth of my second goddaughter in July. As for my own health, it remained robust. And I did what I could to keep it that way by getting my first Moderna monovalent booster, this time at my local CVS. I also continued my workouts without interruption.

As my August stay in Provincetown came to a close, my thoughts began turning to finally catching up with Austin in Denver. My cousin in Sedona, Arizona, also wanted me to visit her, so in October, I left for both destinations with Denver up first.

Austin met me outside my hotel, and we drove in his SUV to 3030 Downing Street in the RiNo neighborhood for my first in-person Apex inspection. It was late morning so the gym was fairly quiet. On one hand, I was definitely impressed with the overall facility and the equipment. The feel was professional and inviting. But I was also alarmed to see that parts of the gym remained cordoned off and unfinished, including the boxing studio. The administrative office was in sorry shape, bathrooms were not in tiptop condition, and some of the drop-ceiling tiles had been removed, probably to facilitate electrical and plumbing work that still needed to be finished.

I didn't want to seem critical or discouraging so I refrained from sharing my first impressions—both positive and otherwise—and we left for lunch at one of RiNo's hip eateries. Over a humongous salad, Austin shared his frustration with the lack of progress in completing the facility. Constant bickering among the landlord, the contractors and Austin had impeded the completion of the gym. Austin was working with an attorney, an Apex member— but she seemed to have made little if any headway in resolving the unfinished state of affairs. I volunteered to be part of a phone conversation with her later that day, but once that was over, I had no sense that she or anyone else was going to move things forward. It was all very frustrating, both for me and of course for Austin.

The next afternoon, I put the best spin on the previous day's events. I traveled once more to the gym and this time found it overflowing with enthusiastic members. The place was hopping— all the more reason to bewail the Gordian knot that was Apex Human Performance.

That evening, I took Austin and his girlfriend out to Ruth's Chris Steak House in downtown Denver. We had a really nice dinner, and reminisced about our year together in Boston. Later, we returned to Apex where I finally got to meet frisky Oakley. Dog and I bonded quickly, then Austin drove me back to my hotel, where we said our farewells. The next morning I departed by plane for Sedona.

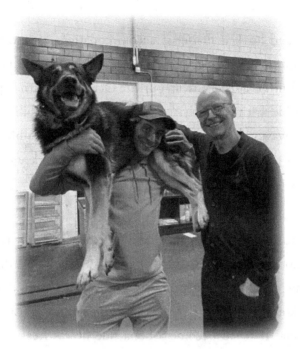

Reunion in Denver

My cousin had told me she was attracted to Sedona after several vacations there because of the unique red and auburn colors that the background landscapes revealed. I totally agreed. The hues were utterly amazing, and I reveled in the mountain and rock-formation tones on my late morning hike not too far from her gorgeous home.

The next day, we traveled to the Grand Canyon, a national treasure I had never seen before.

We had booked first-class accommodations on the historic *Grand Canyon Railway,* another tip of the hat to my train-buff enthusiasm. As a special treat, our late October sojourn happened to coincide with an early-season snowstorm. Visibility at the Canyon was brief, but spectacular. I could not have been more in awe of the sights I beheld. I decided then and there to return someday—a goal I still must honor.

I returned to Boston on Friday, October 15, and resumed my sessions with Pete the following Tuesday. Not that they had been interrupted by my trip out west. I managed to allot time for workouts both at my Denver hotel and at my cousin's place in Sedona. If I had become a bona fide fitness freak, I would revel in my addiction, both in Boston and beyond. And I found it a distinct pleasure to take Pete along for the ride thanks to cellphones and WiFi—our 21st-century magic tools.

Chapter Sixteen

"PICKY, PICKY, PICKY"

B ack in Boston that fall, I resumed my usual calendar of events, which included not only exercise activities, but musical ones as well. I had for some time fancied myself a student of the harpsichord, the keyboard precursor to the piano, whose strings are plucked instead of hammered. That year I learned Johann Sebastian Bach's *French Suite Number 5 in G major,* and on November 5, I completed a video of all the pieces with a recording of its last movement, a French dance called a gigue. Aside from my workouts, I considered playing the entire suite one of my proudest (and more athletic) achievements in retirement.

I also resumed my patronage of the Boston Symphony and attended chamber music recitals at the Harvard Musical Association on Beacon Hill. If my plate was full, I was glad for it, as I had no use for an inert life. At seventy-one, I remained as eager as ever to remain in the game.

And that also meant returning to Florida for an extended winter stay in South Beach. My hope was to return to the familiar Decoplage, and I got in touch with my chatty real estate agent with whom I had previously worked to secure month-long leases there. Happy to hear from me again, she told me that demand was greater than ever, thanks to the countrywide reopening, and prices had gone up a tad. In fact, my old apartment had already been booked by someone else, but another unit on a higher floor was still available. She mentioned that it had been totally renovated and was available for a minimum two-months stay of $20,000.

Sticker shock would be an understatement. I had paid no more than $5,000 per month in the past, and there was no way I was going to shell out $20,000 for an apartment, however luxurious the remodeling. Still, I wanted desperately to abandon New England for the winter, so for the first time, I considered the option of buying a condo. Surely its monthly costs, I reasoned, wouldn't approach $10,000—especially if I went in on this with a partner and without a mortgage.

I got in touch with the friend who had stayed with me at the Decoplage in previous years, and we agreed to start searching. By then I had become expert at arranging trips around my scheduled sessions with Pete on Tuesdays and Thursdays, so on Friday, November 12, we left on a five-day home hunting expedition.

My first thoughts were to secure something on Collins Avenue. But condos were scarce on this side of town as the surfeit of hotels attested. Moreover, most oceanfront properties in that neighborhood seemed reserved for short stays. Our new real estate broker suggested that we focus our search on the bay side of the island. I had never spent much time there except for a couple of restaurant visits, but I liked the idea of a quieter residential space, so for the next three days, we scoured units west of Alton Road on West Avenue and Bay Road.

House hunting is an exhausting affair, both physically and mentally. And after three days of searching, everything we had seen became one giant blur in my mind. Fortunately, I had taken notes and we had our broker's crib sheets. We saw places with fantastic views of the Atlantic and others of Biscayne Bay. One even boasted views of both, but the layout was so bizarre that it failed to survive our cut list. Another was so depressing that we never made it past the foyer.

And then there was the two-bedroom condo occupied by three humans, six cats and one dog. Or maybe it was two dogs, hard to tell. As much as I tried to imagine the apartment without the animals, I just couldn't bring myself to consider it a viable prospect. We left on Wednesday afternoon, November 17, having failed to identify even one unit we would consider bidding on.

The next day I met Pete back at my Boston apartment building's fitness center. I reported on my trip and its lack of results. He had been to Miami Beach recently, so he knew the lay of the land. We briefly talked about the challenges I was facing. But none of this kept us from the main matter at hand as he coached me in his signature blend of new and old routines.

Among the latter were cable V bar back rows. I distinctly recalled doing these in my early days with Austin at Equinox, albeit in a seated position. A V bar handle was attached to a cable machine and I slowly pulled the bar to my chest. Various weights could be added or subtracted. In my fitness center I did the rows in a standing position with the cable in high or low mode. However they're done, the trick is always to keep your back in a neutral position.

Ditto for another routine we did that afternoon—the evocatively named goblet squats. (I may have done these at Equinox, too, but I can't be certain.) A goblet squat required me to hold a kettlebell or a dumbbell in front of my chest—hence the goblet shape. I would then squat as deeply as possible, which wasn't easy. The squat itself worked the glutes and quadriceps, and the trick—as I shortly found out—was to descend while keeping the bell firmly on my chest without collapsing into the dreaded catlike spinal position. If I even showed a hint of the feline, Pete would "Quasimodo" me back into proper alignment.

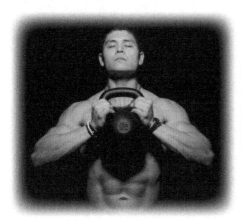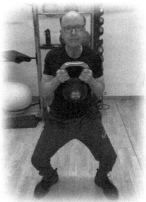

Goblet squats with Pete demonstrating a proper
grip and me struggling to stay neutral

Truth to tell, I never really got used to these verbal blandishments; they often came fast and furious. But I knew what they meant—that Pete wanted me to be as strict about form as I was about working hard. After a while, I came up with a regular rejoinder, which pleased me no end and which Pete found very funny. As he invoked once more the hunchback of Notre Dame, I sarcastically responded, "Picky, picky, picky." To this day, he can't help laughing whenever I invoke my trademark catchphrase.

Chapter Seventeen

YEAR-END APPRAISALS

Several days after my return, I got a call from my real estate agent. A two-bedroom condo had just been placed on the market in the Mirador 1000, the building with the cats-and-dogs unit. In fact, it was in the same tier, only higher and with a better view of the Atlantic on the eastern horizon. Would I be interested in a FaceTime appointment to see it?

Animals aside, I liked the unit we had visited. The building appeared well maintained; it had a spacious swimming pool, and most important for me, a large fitness center. It was also just a block away from Whole Foods, a considerable asset since I had no desire to saddle myself in Florida with a car and its attendant costs. Besides, I was supposed to be walking as much as possible, and that meant moving beyond brief strolls for groceries. The building's location on Tenth Street was ideally suited both for sauntering down to South Pointe and making northbound trips to Lincoln Mall and beyond.

On FaceTime, the condo looked presentable. The kitchen and the two bathrooms were out of date, so that would factor into my decision if we made an offer—and for how much. But the overall feel was welcoming, and the views of the ocean from the living room and balcony were exceptional. As we concluded the call, I consulted with my prospective co-owner, and we decided to make an offer: fifteen-thousand dollars below the asking price.

Lo and behold, in twenty-four hours, the offer was accepted. It seemed odd buying a property without actually having stepped foot inside it. I was also taken aback by the rapidity of the seller's response, given the many months it took to sell my home in Boston. But I knew that there could still be delays before the title was transferred. I also wanted to be physically present for the building inspection, which I considered mandatory. I quickly got in touch with Pete, moved my next session up from Tuesday to Monday, and on December 14, flew to Miami International for a whirlwind twenty-four hour stay—just three weeks since my departure. Without missing a beat, I kept my regular appointment back in Boston with Pete on Thursday the 16th.

By year's end, my routine for working out had largely returned to its pre-Pandemic rhythms—uninterrupted by virtual sessions, aside from relatively brief forays to New York. Twice weekly, Pete walked fifteen minutes from downtown Boston to my apartment building in the West End. (I paid a modest premium for this personal service). On off-Pete days, I went downstairs to the fitness center, also twice a week—though sometimes three, depending on my energy level and mood—and spent an hour on endurance and intensity exercises. These involved my Holy Trinity of machines: the StairMaster, the rowing machine and the elliptical.

If I was on the elliptical, I watched videos of hikes though Bryce Canyon National Park, Grand Teton and other out-West venues. Sometimes I'd get dizzy following the vertiginous trails and would turn off the screen to focus on the blank wall in front of me. My typical difficulty level was seven out of twenty— maybe just below a Goldilocks mean. But I wasn't as young as Goldilocks, either!

With rowing, I emphasized spurts over endurance. I usually did twenty seconds of high intensity movements followed by forty seconds in slow motion. I repeated this pattern over ten minutes. All things considered, I deemed the results fine, if not sensational.

Once I decided to embrace it—you may recall I originally had anxiety over mounting and dismounting—the StairMaster presented fewer hurdles than I might have expected. Having lived in a four-story walk up for forty years, I was used to climbing stairs. I quickly went from thirty to forty-five to sixty minute periods. I even moved my body sideways—an unorthodox position I had observed a fit young woman perform, though I would not recommend it for most folks my age. I'd initially go nonstop no matter the length of time, pausing only for a few quick gulps of water from my thermos. In later sessions, I stopped after fifteen to twenty minutes to better catch my breath and drink more water—a prescription that Pete constantly stressed—before resuming the climb for the rest of my allotted time.

As was the case at Equinox, I avoided treadmills. I had seen more people jeopardizing their body parts on these machines, pounding their feet into the running belts and risking knee blowouts. Treadmills are probably better than ellipticals for losing pounds, but I just felt that their risks outweighed the rewards.

—ɯ—

With winter's onset, Covid protocols still remained in place. I wiped all the gym equipment both before and after each use. Masking was still de rigueur, though I noticed more and more persons slipping their masks off for heavy workouts, like I had done at Equinox.

Also as at Equinox, Pete and I got to observe and get to know some of the fitness center's regulars. Our favorite was a Korean War Navy veteran who looked younger than his eighty-eight years. He served as an inspiration for both of us, and reminded me that there is no mandatory retirement age for working out.

On the other side of the "respect spectrum" was the Spritzer, a gentleman with what could only be dubbed as hyper-perspiration syndrome. Now, no one can help how much or how little they spritz—I'm already on record as identifying as a low-sweat case— but this guy left prodigious pools below every machine he used. And he never mopped up after himself! I felt badly for the cleaners that had to cope with his surfeit of wetness.

Hardly anyone considered 2021 to be a banner year. Stop, make that no one. I recall people throughout 2021 confessing that they never imagined it could be worse than 2020. Choosing between the two was a tough call. And yet, one had reason to be sanguine about 2022. There were signs that the battle against the coronavirus was turning in our favor. The new administration in Washington had botched the withdrawal from Afghanistan, but it also had embarked in November on a string of bipartisan legislative victories. Some even ventured the opinion that the grownups were back in charge. That, too, may have been optimistic.

Chapter Eighteen
STRESSED OUT

On January 1, I invited my five-month old goddaughter, her brother and their parents to my home for a traditional roast turkey dinner with all the usual trimmings. It was their first visit anywhere as a family since her birth, and I was honored to be their host. She was the perfect guest, never cried or said boo. If anything, she seemed overly demure—unlike her rambunctious older sibling, who noodled on the harpsichord before crashing into my Christmas tree and nearly toppling it over. A good time was had by all.

The first month of the year typically contained its fair share of doctors' visits and 2022 was no exception. First up on January 12 was a virtual trip via telemedicine to my cardiologist at Massachusetts General Hospital. Nothing unusual there, though I was urged again to cut down on the alcohol and caffeine. His post-visit notes revealed that I confessed to four or five cups of coffee in the morning and two to three alcoholic drinks at night. I thought that was unusually candid of me.

Next stop was dermatology on the 18th. Again, no surprises, though numerous actinic keratosis lesions on my scalp had prompted me to make this visit in advance of my previously scheduled appointment. Two days later I was in the dental hygienist's chair for my thrice-yearly cleaning. Finally, on the 26th, I returned to my primary care physician for my annual senior's wellness visit.

Here again, test results proved unexceptional and consistent with the prior year's. My blood pressure was 134/78. Pulse was 82. Weight was 153 pounds. My temperature recorded at 96.9–even lower than in 2021; I attributed my aversion to winter to this chronic state of under heating. But best of all for my vanity's sake was her written comment that, with regard to my appearance, "He is well-developed." I must say that made my day.

There was one troubling cause for concern, and that did not relate to me, but to my doctor. I asked her how she was doing and she replied ominously, "hanging in there." I could tell just from her tone that the past year had taken a toll on her. We talked a little about her practice, the deaths of her patients from the virus, and for a few moments, I felt like a physician ministering to his patient. I left that morning and knew that I would not see her again. On August 9, I received her message that "I have made the difficult decision to leave my practice and make a career change, which is the best decision for my family at this time."

In four years, I had churned through three primary care practitioners—and now I would need a fourth. For me, this turnstile of physicians gave lie to the notion that PCPs knew their patients and their needs well enough to better care for them over time, referring them only when necessary to specialists for further treatments. In my experience, however caring PCPs may be (and one of mine was seriously not), they were basically functionary-gatekeepers onto a dysfunctional healthcare universe. I worried about how this sorry state of affairs was adversely impacting those of my peers and friends who were in declining mental or physical shape.

In February, I began developing dental problems that had gone undiagnosed and unaddressed during Covid shutdowns in 2020 and 2021. First up was growing sensitivity and pain in the gum around a lower left molar. I scheduled a visit with a periodontist, who told me the problem was with a tooth, not the gums, and I probably needed root canal work. I dutifully signed up for a trip to an endodontist, who performed only my second such procedure. I then returned to my regular dentist who salvaged the old crown atop the root, thereby saving me a couple thousand dollars.

I would not save the money for long. Just as I was recovering from my second root canal, the molar directly above the lower crown began causing identical pain and discomfort. I couldn't believe my bad fortune. My endodontist speculated that tooth grinding had increased among his patients during the past two years due to stress caused by Covid and the shutdowns. Basically, my teeth had suffered the same fate as my feet.

—∞—

Stress was also accruing from delays in our condo purchase. The seller had neglected to confirm in 2018 that his attorney had filed the paperwork required to have a deceased co-owner's name removed from the title. Caveat emptor: never assume that legal work is done just because you ask a lawyer to do it. Basically we and the seller were in title limbo until this mess was addressed. As the months dragged on, I resigned myself to the irritating fact that I would not be spending much time in Florida this winter after all.

Finally, on March 16, the closing was scheduled. I never met the seller as our communiqués—always through our respective real estate agents and attorneys—had grown increasingly testy and tense since December. Nonetheless, we were delighted to close— however late in the game—and on March 23, my co-owner and I flew to Florida to inspect our freshly-acquired premises for the first time in the flesh.

Without furnishings, we had to stay once more at a hotel. I was fine with that since our principal purpose for the trip to South Beach was to meet the contractor responsible for renovating the bathrooms and kitchen. Having accomplished this objective, we left for Fort Lauderdale on Saturday, March 26, to join a family celebration in honor of my aunt's ninetieth birthday.

Everything went pleasantly and smoothly until the Lyft ride I had scheduled for March 28, which entailed a short trip to Amtrak's Fort Lauderdale station; from there we would board the northbound *Silver Star* about fifteen minutes past noon. I had confirmed a pickup for an hour before, and the driver arrived right on time. He was a congenial senior, a recent emigré from Eastern Europe, he confided. As we departed, my confidence in him sapped quickly as I observed his challenges in programming the GPS. His driving wasn't much better, and my stress levels rose with each passing moment. As we approached the train station on our right, I could palpably sense that he hadn't a clue where he was or when to turn. I shouted "Turn right!" but it was too late as he drove onto the overpass for Interstate 95.

Then in an extraordinary act of incompetence—and against my entreaties—he decided to turn onto the highway and head south toward Miami to make a U-turn. I knew how far we were from the next exit and my heart sank in the sure knowledge that we would never make it back in time to board the *Silver Star*.

I was wrong. We did make it back with about three minutes to spare as the driver profusely apologized for his multiple blunders.

I couldn't bring myself to tip him or report him, for fear that he might lose a job he obviously needed. We boarded the train and I spent the next hour drawing on all my Yoga-learned techniques to lower my blood pressure below stroke-inducing levels.

Chapter Nineteen
TRAIN FOR LIFE

With the new year still in its infancy, both Pete and Austin made tweaks to their careers. Pete expanded his commitment to working with seniors by becoming a vetted personal-trainer provider for Beacon Hill Village, a members-led nonprofit that provides older adults with the resources and information they need "to optimize choices for successful, healthy aging." His Instagram account, Pete's Peak Performance, now bore the epigram "Don't just train for today. Train for Life." My title for this memoir must have been inspired by Pete's creed, though I can't say that I consciously poached it from him.

Meanwhile, in Denver, Austin made the tough decision to shutter Apex Human Performance. He had given it his best shot, but the economics remained as daunting as ever. He moved much of his old equipment to a new building with lower rent at 4700 Brighton Road north of RiNo, and reopened his new gym with the title Apex Performance Training. The travel time between the two sites was no more than about twenty minutes by car, and some of his clients continued at the new space. But it remained an open question as to whether this venue or any other for that matter was commercially viable.

—⟋⟍—

In June I journeyed once again to New York for my fiftieth college reunion at Queens College's spring commencement. Four years before, I had attended my high school fiftieth, which was somewhat disappointing both in turnout and by virtue of its location far from the high school itself. Still, I had enjoyed myself and even saw some schoolmates whom I had known since fifth grade. For the college reunion, I got permission to wear my Yale Ph.D. hood and gown. But I wanted to travel lightly so I left the bulky gown—and it's three-striped "Doctor" sleeves—behind.

As we gathered for the commencement, I borrowed a regular undergraduate gown from our host party and assembled with my fellow classmates of 1972. We would be close to the head of the procession and just behind a far smaller contingent of older alums. As we were ushered through the outdoor throng of undergraduates and their families, I heard a few "bravos" and "hurrays" coming from the crowd followed by a loud round of applause. I couldn't figure out what was going on—until it dawned on me: my peers and I were being acclaimed for being alive! We geezers had survived all the plagues of the past fifty years, and we were still ticking. I confess that I experienced the tributes with mixed emotions. I was touched by the applauders' sincerity, but I also felt mildly annoyed at being deemed "old." I had felt the same ambivalence the first time someone offered me a seat on the subway. It was a feeling I would have to get used to with each passing year.

———✳———

Having traveled solo for the home inspection at the Mirador 1000 in November, I decided to stay in Boston when my co-owner flew back to Miami in July. Furniture and fixtures were arriving almost daily, and his job was to make certain that all the items were delivered safe and sound. He also hired assemblers—we used to call them handymen—to put everything together. I kept a running tab on the countries of origin: the rugs came from India and Iran. The boomerang coffee tables were Canadian. The sectional sofa was Mexican and the really comfortable resin wicker side chairs were Indonesian. It was a veritable United Nations of furnishings.

Consonant with our ages, we were largely inspired by mid-fifties retro styles. The capstone of this project was a dinette set of table and chairs newly manufactured in the U.S.A.—West Virginia to be precise—that evoked a bygone era of Formica countertops and Naugahyde seat cushions. I was less attached to this aesthetic than my condo partner, but I must say that the dinette set made a striking impression on me the first time I saw it.

While furniture arrived in South Beach, I traveled to a family reunion in Tennessee. In 1972 my oldest cousin had asked me to be her daughter's godfather. I had never taken on this role before, and being eager to do something different and new, I accepted. In the intervening years, I turned out to be a terrible godfather and had barely managed to stay in touch with my godchild. So, when she asked me to join her to celebrate her fortieth wedding anniversary—I had never even met her husband and children—I was determined to attend.

My goddaughter's mother had died some years before, so I called her sister—also the godmother—to plan our trip together. We arranged to meet at Philadelphia International Airport, where I was scheduled to change flights, and then travel jointly to Knoxville. It was also a reunion for the two of us, since I hadn't seen my cousin since her older daughter's wedding almost two decades ago.

The morning after our check-in at the Hilton Knoxville Airport Hotel, our goddaughter met us for the short car trip to her home in Alcoa. The three of us had a lot of catching up to do, but I also got to meet other relatives who had only been names to me until then. I liked them; they were "salt of the earth," as we used to say. I struck up a conversation with my goddaughter's son and we discovered a shared passion for film. I told him to check out John Waters' 1974 cult classic Female Trouble, which I consider one of the all-time great American films.

My favorite encounter was with a young man celebrating his

sixth birthday. I figured out that he was my first cousin, three-times removed—yet another measure of my growing longevity. I gave him a Bluejay Transform police car with remote control. It must have occupied his undivided attention for at least ninety seconds.

The next day, my cousin and I left together for our respective hometowns. At the airport, we agreed that we had made the right decision to make the journey; we even had a good time. We embraced, kissed each other goodbye, and went our separate ways.

Only on our return would we discover that both of us had acquired stuffed noses.

Chapter Twenty

QUARANTINE

I decided to get tested only because of my recent travel. The sole symptom that I exhibited was slight nasal congestion—the kind I had experienced after drinking a glass of white wine in my twenties. I had worn masks in the airports and on the planes. And most of my time in Knoxville and Alcoa had been spent outdoors. So I was mildly surprised when my home test revealed the dreaded double lines.

I called my cousin to check on her condition. She said she had come down with a cold. I told her to get tested. The next day, she called back to say that she too had tested positive. She had already gotten in touch with our goddaughter, who reported that just about everyone at the family reunion was now in the same boat. So much for socializing in the Great Outdoors.

My next step was to cancel a dinner date at Deuxave, a Back Bay French restaurant, for Wednesday, July 27. That hurt, since two friends were planning to pick up the tab. My main concern, however, was for the status of my upcoming trip to the Cape, which was less than two weeks away. While fretting over that uncertainty, I had to call Pete and cancel our live workouts. Neither of us was happy with this state of affairs, and for the next couple of weeks, I returned to my living room for our first virtual sessions there in nearly two years.

I had received my latest Moderna booster shot three months earlier on April 22. My current condition remained mild. In fact, I had no symptoms at all (aside from the stuffy nose), and I attributed this not to luck, but to the vaccine. The problem was that I kept testing positive. With August approaching, my forthcoming stay in Provincetown was beginning to look increasingly dicey.

Due to my positive status, I ventured out only to get food and the like, and I was always masked. But I also hosted a friend up from New York, keeping six feet from him while remaining masked whenever he was in my apartment with me. He stayed a couple of nights, and remained negative. And yet, I still tested positive. I have a younger friend who told me that his parents had tested positive for over two weeks. I was not at all happy to hear this.

I decided then to go online and do some research. Various studies had shown that one could test positive for more than two weeks—especially the older one was—but that the probability of passing the virus on to someone else dropped markedly after five to seven days. This was all I needed to know. My trip to Provincetown would proceed according to plan, and I kept my reservations for dinner at my three favorite restaurants: The Mews, The Red Inn, and Victor's. "Foine doining," as some New Yorkers say, would go forward, after all.

—m—

In years past, I had fancied dividing my stays on the Cape into active and passive weeks. A week of cycling and climbing to the top of the Pilgrim Monument, 350 feet above sea level, qualified as active. Playing cribbage and drinking cocktails at Victor's with my women friends definitely was passive. August 2022 would be more active than usual—though it had its fair share of wine and spirits. Provincetown is a walker's paradise, and I took plenty of power walks, pausing only occasionally to guess the names of the local flowers.

I also traversed the breakwater in the bay again, even though I had just done that the previous summer and usually took a year off between these hikes. On that 2021 outing, I recalled thinking that this might be my last year of rock jumping; but as I approached the lighthouse, a fellow hiker stopped to talk. He mentioned that he was eighty-two and that I had at least another ten years of rock jumping ahead of me. I suspect I was in good part honoring his faith in me by returning to the rocks in 2022.

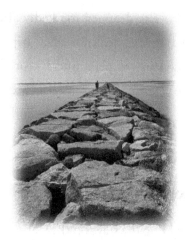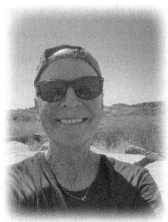

On the breakwater in Provincetown

As usual, my training sessions with Pete did not take a holiday. I brought along my yellow, red and green bands and I worked out in the living room, despite its snug dimensions. He and I had become expert at making the most out of our time together and we weren't about to let diminutive quarters get in our way.

I didn't go swimming. In fact, it had been years since I swam on the Cape, largely because the water temperature is so unpalatable—on the ocean side at Race Point especially, though I remember once swimming in 58 degrees on the bay side at Herring Cove. It was that same summer, some twenty years ago, that I was attacked by a swarm of jellyfish. The older I got, the less I was inclined to suffer these indignities, and my swimming today is confined to pools—preferably heated.

—ɯ—

On August 31, I observed the fifth anniversary of my retirement or, as I noted on Facebook, my "next chapter" in the manner of Serena Williams and Anthony Fauci. Alongside my comment, I posted a gym selfie where I look remarkably healthy and fit for a seventy-one year old. It was amazing what five years of working out—not to mention flattering camera angles and lighting—had accomplished.

I briefly returned to the Cape in September for a special reunion. In college I had been mentored by a woman professor of political science. Indeed, she was the first female granted tenure by the department. She had nurtured my interest in American political institutions, and it was she who set me on my course toward seeking a Ph.D. I hadn't seen her in fifty years and when I discovered that she had retired to the historic town of Sandwich, I resolved to see her again.

We had a grand time catching up, recalling old friends while walking on the beach. Now in her eighties, she remained a model for me on how to age gracefully. Recently widowed, she lives by herself in a lovely home filled with mementos of her personal and professional life. (Her career culminated as president of a university in Pennsylvania.) We talked a little about whether she has a support system in place and, indeed, she counts on a couple of friends to help with home repairs and the like.

I realized in that visit that I cared for her more than I knew.

I also saw myself in her, ten years from now, determined to lead a good life on my own as long as possible. In our reunion, she gave me renewed confidence to face my future with enthusiasm and lust for life itself.

Chapter Twenty-One

HOLIDAY FRENZY

October may be the best time to visit Boston. The temperature usually remains moderate and fall foliage in the city peaks typically around the third week of the month. But as soon as November arrives, skies turn grey and can largely remain that way through April.

Not wishing to tempt fate, I had decided to make my escape from the Northeast on Tuesday, November 1. On Friday, October 28, I bade farewell to the Boston Symphony with a matinee performance—the preferred subscription for folks my age— and then joined up at Grill 23 & Bar, a steakhouse in Back Bay, to celebrate a dear friend's retirement at age seventy-four. (How he lasted that long was anyone's guess, including his.) The following Monday, I took Acela down to New York and caught an evening performance of Puccini's *Tosca* at the Metropolitan Opera. The following day, I departed from La Guardia for Miami International.

I arrived at the Mirador 1000 that afternoon for the first time as a home-owning resident. Our contractor had just finished the kitchen and bathroom redoes the week before, and there was considerable cleanup work ahead of me. But aside from that exercise, I wanted to make the acquaintance of my new gym, Prestige Miami Fitness Club, also in the Mirador 1000.

On purchasing the condo, I had been told that Prestige was free to the building's residents—not quite, it turned out. A squabble between our condo association and a master association comprised of three buildings including the Mirador 1000 had provoked a suspension of the free-use agreement, becoming in effect collateral damage to the dispute. I was mildly irked at this discovery, but I remained committed as ever to working out, so I signed up for membership and began paying the monthly dues.

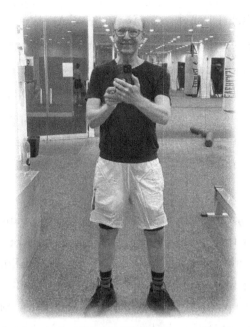

A selfie at Prestige Miami Fitness Club

My first impression of the facility was spacious and LOUD. I was used to ambient noise and canned music through the years, but this was on a different scale altogether. Fortunately, apart from the main floor, there was a smaller room set aside for general exercise and kettlebell classes. And since these classes were few and far between, I made this space my latest workout turf—literally in this case since the room was covered in AstroTurf. I've never understood the love affair between gyms and AstroTurf, since it's murder on your hands and especially your knees.

I continued my Tuesday and Thursday virtual sessions with Pete in the Turf room. And to help with hearing (and to cancel out the noise), I bought my first pair of Apple's AirPods Pro 2 at Pete's recommendation. It was yet another step toward my total immersion in the Apple ecosystem, as I had already profited from several generations of iPhones, iPads and MacBooks. My cardiologist once recommended that I buy the Apple Watch for its robust health and wellness functions, but that purchase has remained on my to-do list.

The funny thing about the AirPods was that I couldn't keep them in my ears. I tried pushing them, twisting them—nothing worked. Exercising with them was futile since they kept falling out. Pete suggested experimenting with the different sizes of silicone tips that came with the package, but whether they were XS, S, M or L made no difference. Pete said he had never experienced this problem himself or with his clients. I wasn't sure what to do—aside from returning the AirPods—so I went to amazon.com and discovered that an entire cottage industry had sprung up to address this problem.

After surveying the territory, I decided to buy AhaStyle anti-slip ear covers, a silicone accessory that you fit over the AirPods. Each cover comes with an appendage that you hook into the auricle or the top outer part of the ear. Getting them on the AirPods is no simple undertaking, and I could imagine lots of people my age giving up trying. Pete and I jokingly dubbed them condoms for the ears since—when used properly—they do the job. I've rarely had the AirPods fall out since buying the covers, but I still must reserve at least a few minutes of prep time to make sure I've placed them on correctly, yet another parallel with prophylactics.

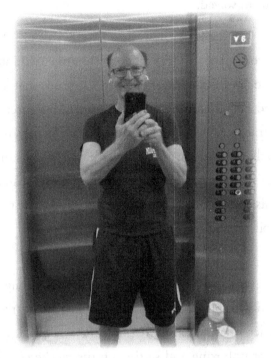

"Condoms for the ears"

On Thursday, December 22, I broke my training schedule with Pete to fly back to Boston for the holidays. Aside from turning on the thermostat, my first order of business was setting up the Christmas tree in my apartment, which I accomplished in record time. In my haste, however, I neglected to test the lights before attaching all the ornaments, and when I plugged the tree in, I discovered that an entire strand of lights had failed. Not one to waste even a minute, I immediately left to purchase a new set at the nearest CVS, which had already placed its holiday items on sale. I scooted back to my tree, plugged in the new lights and voilà, problem solved.

Mind you, all of this transpired within ninety minutes of my arrival at Logan International Airport. I concede that most of my friends and acquaintances would consider this utter madness. And I definitely understand their point. But thanks to my high energy levels and chronic anxiety over leaving things unfinished, I could not help myself. I just had to finish what I had set out to do. (It's this same momentum that has propelled me to complete this memoir as rapidly as possible.)

That evening, I settled into my armchair with a mug of mulled wine spiked with blackberry brandy. I looked at my tree with the same wonder I had felt at Christmastime as a child. I'd already decided that unboxing and setting up the crèche could wait till tomorrow. Perhaps I wasn't as mad as my friends think. I don't recall whether I slept well that night, but with all the travel, work and wine within me, I'd say it was a decent bet to wager on.

The next day, at four PM, ever accommodating Pete Goulet met me to resume our live collaboration. I cannot say that live sessions are superior to virtual workouts. The Apple camera in my iPhone is so exacting that I sometimes have thought that Pete picked up flaws in my movements that might go undetected live.

But as grateful as I am for our virtual partnership, actual training in a shared physical space is its own reward. I shudder for the day when virtual reality and artificial intelligence take us ever further from our defining human identity as social animals.

Chapter Twenty-Two

TAKING STOCK

With the new year, I indulged in the annual ritual for taking stock of my accomplishments, particularly with respect to wellness and health. The most significant improvement I'd noted since my first days with Austin had been a dramatic reduction of chronic low back pain. Pete has credited this to my ongoing exercise regimen and improved core strength. The occasional back spasms have become far less frequent, and my recovery from them more rapid.

Several years ago, I stumbled upon a YouTube channel for physical therapist Jeff Cavaliere's Athlean-X programs. One of these is called How to Fix "Low Back" Pain (Instantly!). It's probably the most important wellness video I've watched. Whenever I have a back flare up, Pete has had me follow the Athlean-X protocol. If you have back problems, I urge you to watch Cavaliere's ten-minute demonstration. You won't regret it, as attested to by the uniformly positive comments from many of the thirty-seven million viewers who've watched him.

I've also been able to maintain my overall strength through a regular program of weightlifting that focuses as much on good form as building power and brawn. Weightlifting is especially important for someone my age since it counters the loss of muscle mass that everyone will experience over time.

Pete has also commented that he's observed improvements in the recovery time I require after a strenuous bout of exercise. High-intensity spurts like a minute of cross-jab shadow boxing don't require a full minute of rest before the next spurt resumes. Also, my tolerance for longer high-intensity exercise has improved. All of this probably speaks to better cardiovascular health. My cardiologist has said that he may place me on a blood thinner like Coumadin once I turn seventy-five. I'm now thinking that he may want to defer that prescription for at least a couple more years.

—⟁—

In taking stock of achievements, I also considered my shortfalls. The holiday season had taken its toll on my weight, which had crept back to 158. I had noted the latest fad for drug-induced weight loss, but I knew that wasn't for me, even if I could get my hands on the injections. In prior years, I had experimented with intermittent fasting—usually eating over eight hours followed by sixteen hours of abstaining, but I didn't feel the results were worth the effort.

I talked with Pete about my pound-creep problem, and he

volunteered a tack that I had never seriously entertained. He suggested I try a low-carb keto diet. I have a friend who had great success with keto, but I had been concerned for her health because of the keto rule to go heavy on fats. Of course, that was just one of many keto rules, so with Pete's blessing, I began reducing my calories and carbs, while eating more protein and fats.

I ate chicken and fish, meats, eggs and salads with scant attention to the globs of salad dressing I added. I abandoned bread, pasta, and ice cream—any desserts, really—which I didn't especially miss. I even restricted my intake of wine at first, preferring to imbibe vodka with its fewer calories. I actually enjoyed not feeling guilty about eating fats. I did miss toast in the morning.

The results were impressive and dramatic; in four weeks, I had lost ten pounds; by the end of March, I was down to 143—a fifteen-pound loss. That had been my goal, and having reached it, I relaxed the near-total ban on carbs. My weight continued to fluctuate between 143 and 147, but I was comfortable within that range—both physically and psychologically. My waistline stabilized at thirty-two inches. I still have my size 31 jeans, and I just may try them on again.

My return to New England over the holidays had not been all that enjoyable due to typically crummy weather throughout my two-week stay. So I was happy to fly back to Florida, where I remained until the end of March. I continued to patronize Prestige Miami Fitness Club, and was delighted to discover that the kerfuffle over membership fees had been resolved in favor of Mirador 1000 residents like me. Somehow, not paying to play made the noise and AstroTurf more palatable.

I traveled on one occasion to West Palm Beach to watch a friend's horse compete in his first derby at Wellington International. I even bought a twenty-four dollar baseball cap on that occasion to protect my head from the blazing sun. (I had my annual photodynamic therapy scheduled for April and knew that even a mild suntan—much less a burn—would mean cancellation of the treatment.)

I also had high hopes for a reunion with Austin around this time, as he was planning to take part in TYR Wodapalooza Miami, a four-day fitness competition involving some of the world's elite athletes. He would be participating in the team divisions along with some of his Denver buddies. We had talked about his staying at my place, though I reminded him that Miami and Miami Beach are two separate cities and that getting from one to the other during morning and evening causeway commutes would not be ideal. Ultimately, he wisely opted to stay in Miami, and we did not reconnect. I was sorry about that.

On a FaceTime call earlier in the year, Austin told me that he had finally decided to close Apex's latest iteration. He had kept the enterprise afloat for five years—about the lifespan for most small businesses. But with that decision, he also determined that he would leave Denver and return to the East Coast. On the car trip down to Miami, he had scouted out a diverse set of prospective locations, finally deciding to put down roots in Raleigh, North Carolina. From a new home there, this "lifestyle and fitness entrepreneur"—as his Instagram page proclaims—continues to push the health and wellness envelope, both in daily workouts and in competitions. He has also taken up the banner of Project 2050 Solar with a mission of creating a fully sustainable planet by the year 2050. If I live to be one-hundred, I'll expect to see that he kept his eyes firmly on that prize.

Chapter Twenty-Three

FIT PHARISEE

Every Lent I eliminate or reduce my alcohol consumption. Years ago, I gave up caffeine and found that far more difficult and challenging; it also left me feeling incredibly testy. For Lent 2023, I decided to limit my drinking to one drink per night, no more. It could be one glass of wine or one martini, but it had to be one and only one. Simple and straightforward, right?

After a week of strictly honoring my intention, I decided I needed to make a tweak: I would divide a martini's contents in half and add a roughly equal amount of water to the vodka or gin, thereby doubling my drinking without doubling the alcohol. Call it martini lite, if you will. I convinced myself I was staying true to my objective, even if a strict legalistic read of my original intent left me feeling like a modern-day Pharisee.

I also enlisted my favorite South Beach bartender in the ruse. Imagine the poor guy having to serve me a martini in one glass, while I poured half of it into another glass, all the while having a spare glass of ice water and yet another glass of dirty rocks also in reserve. I amply tipped him for his service—which was way beyond the call of duty—though I wouldn't be surprised if he secretly considered me one gigantic pest.

Aside from my Lenten devotion, my daily routines in Florida stayed fairly close to the workouts Pete and I had established over the holidays in Boston. I did enjoy the outdoor heat, of course—that was the reason I had decided to winter there in the first place—and I took in as much sun in early mornings and evenings as I thought prudent. My one disappointment was my inability to enjoy the Mirador 1000's swimming pool and deck. In my haste to close on the condo, I glossed over the fine print on the schedule for building repair work. It seemed the epitome of bad fortune to miss out on my first full season of swimming, though I knew my dermatologist would find consolation where I only found frustration.

Throughout the winter months, I was prone to greater introspection than usual. I wanted to know where I was making steady progress, where I was holding steady, and where—if anywhere—I was falling behind. Part of this self-analysis may have had its roots in my decision to write this book. But I also felt that as I grew older, I needed to revisit the yardstick I had previously applied for measuring success.

Some areas of the most pronounced progress were also the most surprising. Despite my past bouts with frozen shoulder, my shoulder mobility and stability were greatly improved since 2017. I was able to press weights overhead and pull cables without any pain at all. If I slept too long on one shoulder or the other, I still felt discomfort, but my overall headway with these ball-and-socket joints was considerable.

I am doubly fortunate never to have suffered knee pain or cartilage degeneration of the knee. I continue to do leg presses with relative ease, though I'm not sure the weight or resistance I can push today is greater than when I started training. Count this as a status quo victory.

One area that resists improving is toe and ankle mobility. On my holiday return to Boston, I revisited my podiatrist and got another round of cortisone shots in my feet. Toe pain continues to constrain my ability to do planks, burpees and squat thrusts, and I have now resigned myself to the prospect that this will continue to be a problem for me down the road.

Pete still has high hopes for improving my ankle mobility so I can do better, deeper squats. I actually never feel pain in my ankles, and suspect that any shortcomings in working these joints is attributable to me favoring my toes over the ankles. It would make sense that this is the case, since I'm always mindful of any movements that might provoke toe pain. My ankle mobility just might be paying the price.

—∞—

While thinking about my own progress and goals, I also began to muse on how trainers measure their professional successes and failures. It occurred to me that I had never asked Pete about his credentials. Massachusetts does not require personal trainers to be certified; nonetheless, most gyms and fitness centers in the Bay State require certification for employment—ditto for Florida. There are a plethora of national certifying entities. I discovered that Pete is certified by the nonprofit American Council on Exercise or ACE, which in turn is accredited by NCCA, the National Commission for Certifying Agencies.

ACE requires that its applicants hold certificates in both CPR and AED—or automatic external defibrillator—techniques. An exam determines initial certification success or failure; those who succeed must then demonstrate sustained competence through continuing education credits and a biennial certification renewal process. As with most certifying and accrediting procedures, the endgame isn't just about setting standards: it's also about establishing barriers to entry and determining who gets to go to the head of the line.

I already knew that Pete pays close attention to client retention and growing his client base. He also has established clear financial goals for himself, and has almost certainly saved and invested far more than the average twenty-nine year old. Even accounting for inflation, it's got to be far more than what I had at his age. Pete lives in and for the present, but he also plans prudently for the future.

Personal trainers have tough schedules. Clients who work often prefer sessions before nine and after five. That can make for really long workdays. Chronic stress and boredom are often-cited causes for trainer burnout. Exhaustion also plays a role. I have never felt that Pete defaults to automatic pilot around me, though he occasionally slips up and calls me by the name of another client he has just seen. He regularly breaks in new routines and tries out fresh approaches. He always remains curious and inquisitive. All of these are positive signs that augur well for his ability to avoid burnout as he enters his thirties and second decade of professional work.

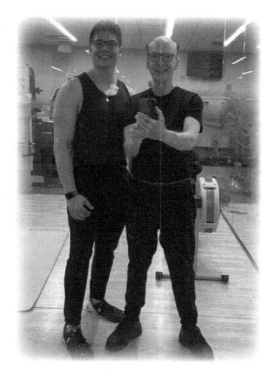

Pete and me

Chapter Twenty-Four

"NO EXCUSES" REDUX

Around Easter, I began experiencing discomfort after multiple dental visits for both a root canal and a crown restoration. Within days, my left cheek had swollen and was tender to the touch. Apparently, an infection had developed near the site of the restoration, which had left a gap between two molars—a perfect breeding ground for bacteria. In an effort to prevent the little buggers from replicating, I was given a two-week prescription for Amoxicillin, the go-to drug for battling gonorrhea and other pestilences. When the medication ran out, I was told, the infection and the inflammation would be gone.

A few days passed and the swelling and tenderness remained—no worse, no better. It was Tuesday, a Pete day, but the last thing on my mind was training. We were scheduled for a 3:30 PM session at the fitness center in my Boston apartment building so nothing could have been more convenient. Still, I felt I had a legitimate case for canceling. I began to muse on the possibility. In my inflamed state, the prospect seemed tempting—even seductive.

Fantasizing about not exercising is an idée fixe for me—it's part and parcel of the overall training experience. Working out is work, after all, and those like me who are old enough to recall Dobie Gillis's beatnik friend Maynard G. Krebs know that we humans often find work allergy-inducing. On the other hand, there are social elements of the experience that I always look forward to. I like the banter with Pete. The fact that he's forty-plus years younger than I am helps me to feel young—or, at least, younger. He keeps me on top of contemporary personalities and events. He has often talked of things about which I know nothing. And I have had the pleasure of introducing him to the likes of Groucho Marx and Jimmy Durante. Pete absolutely loves "Hotch-cha-cha-cha-cha. Everybody wants ta get into da act!"

I finally decided not to cancel. In my gut I knew I wouldn't. Indeed, I've never canceled except once after a bad reaction to the mega-dose seniors flu vaccine. The session went well with no concessions made to my condition. And—happy to say—by our next encounter on the following Thursday, the nasty bacteria were in full retreat.

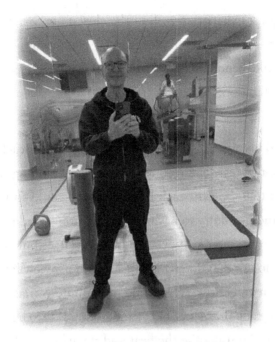

Home in Boston, April 2023

With my mouth restored to normalcy, I went ahead with a previously planned trip to Florida for a two-week stay, punctuated by a two-night stand in Savannah. I had intended to return in order to oversee some plumbing repairs; of course, I renewed acquaintance with my local watering hole, where I finally ordered something stronger than a martini lite. Pete and I also resumed our virtual workouts, this time with an emphasis on using kettlebells—something of a specialty at Prestige Fitness. I did minute-long hip swings with a bell that weighed about thirty-five pounds. Prestige's bells were calibrated in kilograms, so every time Pete asked me to locate a bell of so many pounds, I would have to do a quick calculation to find the closest approximate size in kilograms. I made the blunder once of picking up a heavy bell with a catlike bend to my back. I was promptly "Quasimodo-ed" for that infraction.

As had been the case during my time at South Beach Boxing, Prestige felt awfully hot at times. The air conditioning at Prestige was better than South Beach Boxing's, but I could still count on the heat and humidity to have an impact on my workout. I guess in one sense it's better to exercise in the heat; it burns off more calories, though that doesn't compensate in my view for the extra perspiration and effort. As I've said, my mind invariably wanders to canceling appointments, or at least getting Pete to lighten up on my activities. But despite the heat and my whining, Pete guided me through reasonably invigorating workouts. And as has been the the case since 2017, I always feel much better after a session than I do before.

I returned to Boston on Wednesday, May 24, well-rested and ready for my live workout with Pete the following day. It felt good to be back even if the weather remained unseasonably cool and grey. After forty-plus years, you'd think I would be used to New England's fickle climate, but paying for indoor electric heat as we entered June was like pouring the proverbial salt in the wound.

As you can tell if you've made it this far with me, I am

an evangelist for personal training. But over the past six years, I hadn't succeeded in making any converts. That all changed in June. My seventy-four year old friend and neighbor—whose retirement we celebrated in October—had found little to occupy his time in the ensuing months. I grew concerned as I observed his weight loss and what appeared to be muscle atrophy. His legs especially seemed to grow increasingly spindly. When I went out with him, I would become alarmed that he might fall. (He had already fallen several times in his apartment.)

I explained all of this to Pete, who I thought was ideally qualified to help turn things around. I introduced Pete to my friend, and much to my delight and amazement, they agreed to start training. The first few sessions would be all about balance and floor exercises. I'm happy to say that even after just a few weeks of working together, the improvements in steadiness and confidence were tangible. I have high hopes that these advances will not only be sustained, but will continue to accrue over time. Thank you, Pete Goulet! And thank you again to Austin Rowe for having skillfully launched me on this life-enhancing adventure six years ago.

So please remember: it's never too late to take your first steps. You did it as a toddler and you can do it again. You owe it to yourself above all else. And as I said at the beginning of our journey together in chapter one (it bears repeating), "When all is said and done, keep to your plan. I guarantee, you will not regret it!"

ABOUT THE AUTHOR

David E. Lapin is the author of *The Education of Brainiac: A New Yorker's Quest for the Good Life in the Hub of the Universe* (iUniverse, 2019). Born in the Bronx and raised in Puerto Rico and New York City, Lapin has lived in Boston since 1980. He has served on the boards of the Boston Center for the Arts, the Harvard Musical Association, the National Guild for Community Arts Education, and numerous citizen advisory committees on everything from arts education to air rights development over the Massachusetts Turnpike.

Lapin has also lectured and participated in panels for Berklee College of Music, Longy School of Music of Bard College, the Massachusetts Cultural Council and the New England Conservatory. He has been an advisor to The Learning Project in Boston's Back Bay, Jamaica Plain's Eliot School of Fine Arts, and EdVestors Boston Public Schools Arts Education Initiative. He continues to support Community Music Center of Boston—which he led from 1983 until 2017—as a member of its Corporation. He also chairs Harvard Musical Association's Achievement Awards Committee.

Lapin holds a Ph.D. in political science from Yale University, and has taught at Yale and Cornell. His doctoral dissertation, *No-Growth Democracy*, explores the viability of democratic systems in the absence of economic growth.

Printed in the United States
by Baker & Taylor Publisher Services